Proton Warriors

Surviving Prostate Cancer AND
the Prostate Cancer Industry

Harold H. Dawley Jr., Ph.D.

Wellness Institute/ Self-Help Books
515 W. North St. Pass Christian, MS 39571

Limit of liability and disclaimer of warranty

While care has been taken in writing this book the author and publisher make no claims or warranties in regard to the accuracy or completeness of the information provided in it and specifically disclaim any implied warrantees for any specific purpose. This book, like many books, is not perfect and may contain errors or inaccuracies. The author is not a physician and does not claim any expertise in understanding prostate cancer other than that which comes from having it treated through proton therapy. Nothing in this book is intended to be medical advice. Material appearing here represents opinions offered by a non-medically-trained layperson and should NEVER be interpreted as specific medical advice and must be used only as background information when consulting with a qualified medical professional. The advice and strategies provided may not be suitable to all readers and consultation with a qualified medical professional is recommended when appropriate. It is not the intention of this book to encourage readers to ignore the advice of their physician for doing so may lead to unnecessary health risks. Its primary intention is to encourage its readers to become more informed about prostate cancer and the different treatments for it so that they can make informed decisions in selecting the treatment that best suits their needs.

Acknowledgements

I want to thank the wonderful people who helped me with this book. My wife Linda gets first thanks for her patience and tireless help in editing. Next, to my son Michael who handled the production of this book. Thanks go to my fellow patients who went through treatment with me and completed my surveys. Thanks to Sarah, Shane, Marci, Marilyn and the rest of my treatment staff particularly Tai Lee at the proton therapy Center. I must add that I don't miss the free morning balloons that were part of my proton therapy. Special thanks go to our own talented stand–up comic Henry who kept us laughing as we went through treatment together even though he did steal many of my jokes. To Joe and Marcia, Gary and Pam, Tom and Cindy, Judy and Steve, and Lina and Bob for the enjoyable diners we had together. Thanks go to Bert Vorstman, urologist, for courageously advocating non-invasive treatments of prostate cancer and for writing an introduction to this book. Thanks to my psychologist colleague Joel Block for joining me in writing Appendix A on Erectile Fitness training. My very special thanks go to Ralph Blum, a successful author, who kindly took the time to review this book and write the Foreword.

Harold H. Dawley, Jr., Ph.D.

About the Author

Harold H. Dawley Jr., Ph.D., ABPP, is director of Wellness Institute/Self-Help Books, LLC. He spent twenty years on the staff of the New Orleans Veterans Affairs Medical Center where he served as the Chief of the Psychiatry Service Day Hospital and Day Treatment programs as well as Smoking Control Officer. For over a decade he also held clinical faculty appointments in the Department of Pathology at the Louisiana State University Medical School, the Department of Medicine and the Department of Psychiatry and Neurology at Tulane University School of Medicine, and an adjunct faculty appointment in the Department of Allied Sciences at Tulane University School of Public Health and Tropical Medicine. Recipient of the Outstanding Psychologist of the Year award from the Louisiana Psychological Association and the Distinguished Service Award from the Division of Psychologists in Public Service of the American Psychological Association (APA) and other awards and honors for his clinical, public service and research work, Dr. Dawley was elected a Fellow of the APA. He is a Past President of the APA Division of Psychologists in Public Service and is also a Past President of the National Association of Veterans Affairs Psychologists. He achieved status as an internationally recognized expert on smoking cessation and has authored five books and seventy articles. His most popular publications include *Friendship—How To Make and Keep Friends*, (Prentice-Hall) a book available both in English and French and *Freedom From Fear* (Tempo Books). He is married and his wife, Linda, has a Ph.D. in education.

About the Publisher

Wellness Institute/Self-Help Books, LLC was one of the first digital self-help publishers and has published over 100 self-help books in the last 14 years. Its authors are mainly Ph.D. and M.D. level mental health professionals and among them were seven who had previously had one or more best selling self-help books. Its books are printed under the Imprint Selfhelpbooks.com which is also the name of its website.

SelfHelpBooks.com

What Readers Are Saying About This Book

"An excellent commentary conveying the emotional reaction upon hearing the words *'you have prostate cancer.'* It explains why most, if not all, of us who have gone through proton therapy selected this treatment tailored to our specific needs. The ease of the treatment with its minimal risk of side effects combined with the knowledge, professionalism, and warmth of M.D. Anderson's physicians, technicians, and support staff made this treatment a surprising experience focused on patient camaraderie instead of being self-centered with thoughts of cancer. Dr. Harold Dawley has accurately captured the humor, dressing room antics, and social bonding that happened in our treatment as we became 'proton warriors' facing our common threat of prostate cancer. This book is a must read for any man who hears the words, *'you have prostate cancer'"*.

Lew Brown, Montgomery, TX (former resident of Houston, native Tennessean, and U.S. Marine).

"This book is a winner! Its important warning to men about the dangers of the prostate cancer industry makes it a book whose time has come. Dr. Dawley does a superb job making men aware of these dangers as well as providing a clear understanding of the advantages of the proton therapy treatment of prostate cancer."

Herb Goldberg, Ph.D., author of bestseller *The Hazards of Being Male*.

"Great book! Tells men exactly what to expect in going through proton therapy and warns them about the dangers of the prostate cancer industry."

Richard Trevino, Spring 2011, M.D.
Anderson proton therapy patient, San Antonio, Texas

"Well researched and well written book with a good mixture of the personal and the medical information men will find worth reading as they decide what to do about their prostate cancer."

M. E. Goodrich, Dr. Sci Hyg, Ph.D.

"Great book!!! The Chapter relating to the 'prostate cancer business' was most interesting and insightful. This book should be a wonderful resource for any man in the process of making decisions about his prostate cancer."

Peter Balsamo, Ph.D., 2011 Proton
therapy patient from University of
Florida Proton Therapy Center.

"Valuable resource men can turn to as they decide what to do about their prostate cancer."

Albert Miller, M.D., Chicago, IL

"Proton Bob started the ball rolling but this is a great book. All newly diagnosed PCa patients should read it carefully. I love the analogy of the wolf with the sheep and using a rifle (proton) vs. a shotgun (photon) to kill it. This book correctly states the key factor to consider is 'side effects', especially when cure rates are comparable. Yes, proton treatment costs more but what is your good health worth?"

Douglas A Palecek, Oshkosh,
Wisconsin. Completed proton therapy
at the CDH Procure Proton Center in
Warrenville, IL in March 2012.

"This book is a delightful and informative read and does a great job of capturing the emotions involved when someone learns they have cancer. Although my experience with my urologist was mostly positive, many of the other patients who went through treatment with Harold and me at M.D. Anderson reported their urologist tried to pressure them into taking treatment from them or an associate. Credit goes to Harold for bringing attention to some of the problems associated with the way prostate cancer is treated. I encourage any man who recently discovered he has prostate cancer to read this excellent book.

Tom Buchanan, Lubbock, Texas, and a fellow Proton Warrior"

Dedication

To the pioneering efforts of Bob Marckini (Brotherhood of the Balloon – ProtonBOB.com) and Joe Landry (ProtonPals.net), two men to whom we owe so much in the battle of prostate cancer.

"The nearly 240,000 in the United States who will learn they have prostate cancer this year have one more thing to worry about: Are their doctors making treatment decisions on the basis of money as much as medicine."

Stephanie Saul, *Profit and Question on Prostate Cancer Therapy*
The New York Times, 2-1-06.

Foreword

Shortly after being diagnosed with prostate cancer, Harold Dawley discovered what many of us who are similarly diagnosed discover, that selecting a treatment that best meets our needs is a journey fraught with risks. The words "You have prostate cancer" leave us shocked, confused and vulnerable to exploitation. It is a dangerous period, one in which, filled with fear, we have to make some of the most important decisions of our lives.

Instead of relying solely on the recommendations of the diagnosing urologist, Dawley did what I and a growing number of other men do—he sought second and third opinions and researched different treatments and their side effects. More important, Dawley sought treatment that would result in the highest quality of life. Far too many men are steered into surgery where they face the very real risk of incontinence and erectile dysfunction. Dawley selected proton therapy. *Proton Warriors – Surviving Prostate Cancer AND the Prostate Cancer Industry* is a compelling account of his surprisingly rewarding experience going through this prostate cancer treatment.

Many of the men going through treatment with Dawley reported negative experiences with the urologists who diagnosed their prostate cancer. A number of them reported feeling pressured to select a treatment the urologist or an associate provided. This experience led him to learn about the multibillion dollar "Prostate Cancer Industry" which he describes as a growing part of the huge medical industrial complex responsible for much of the growing over-treatment and soaring costs of health care today. He goes on to cite articles in leading newspapers such as *The Wall Street Journal, The New York Times* and *The Washington Post,* some of which were critical of "physician self referral" while others raised questions about the serious money at stake and the competition among different treatment providers.

Almost a half-million men in the United States and Europe are annually diagnosed with prostate cancer. Many of these men believe that they are about to die. They don't realize that prostate cancer is different from other cancers. In reality, only about one out of seven men with the disease—perhaps 15%—are actually at risk. Regrettably, many of these men receive treatment they either don't need, or treatment with the risks of severe side effects, when equally effective and less-invasive treatments with fewer side effects are available.

Dawley provides a provocative look from a patient's perspective at how prostate cancer is treated today. He warns men of the dangers inherent in surgical treatment, and emphasizes the importance of making their own informed decisions. This book is well worth reading by any man newly diagnosed with prostate cancer.

Ralph H. Blum, Co-author, *Invasion of the Prostate Snatchers*

An Urologist's View of This Book

As a psychologist and a prostate cancer sufferer, unlike many men, Harold did not panic when diagnosed with his illness. Instead, he empowered himself with knowledge about prostate cancer. Very early in his studies he realized that most of the information available on the treatment of prostate cancer was a veritable soup of half-truths and misinformation, especially concerning the radical surgical/robotic treatment modality. Because he discovered that surgery had a high risk for serious complications and negative quality of life issues, he focused on treatment options that were equally effective but with fewer of the bad side effects. His search led him to one such treatment, a relatively new form of radiation called proton therapy.

Harold shares his journey through proton therapy from interacting with his doctors, treatment staff, and other patients to resuming his life. He reveals the anxiety all men have when told they have prostate cancer. But, more importantly, he shares the surprising degree of pleasure and enjoyment he experienced going through daily treatment with a large number of other men who became his friends. Since sexual problems are a major issue in the treatment of prostate cancer, Harold, along with another psychologist-colleague who is an expert in sex therapy, provide the best guide I have encountered on what men can do to minimize this risk when they receive prostate cancer treatment.

I highly recommend that any man with prostate cancer first read this excellent book before considering treatment such as surgery/robotics. There ARE better, less invasive alternatives to surgery that are equally effective but with less risk for serious permanent complications.

Bert Vorstman MD, MS, FAAP, FRACS, FACS, Prostate Cancer Specialist, Florida Urological Associates, Coral Springs, FL

Table of Contents

Foreword

Urologist's Review of This Book

Chapter One

Prostate Cancer Treatment Today

"My life will never be as great as it was before surgery four years ago. Incontinence is a daily battle. As for intercourse, I now know what a eunuch must feel like – not much. I regret having the surgery,"
E-mail response to a NPT Show
on prostate cancer surgery. [1]

Prostate Cancer Treatment Side Effects

Every night a growing number of American men go to sleep wearing a diaper to control their urinary incontinence. During the day their diaper is replaced with small pads designed to catch and hold the urine escaping from their bladder. Many more men have foregone the sexual enjoyment they have known for much of their lives. Still others experience rectal and other problems. What all of these men have in common are the side effects from having undergone treatment for prostate cancer. It strikes one out of every six of us and is the second cause of our death from cancer with over 200,000 new cases diagnosed annually. Unfortunately, once they are diagnosed with prostate cancer many men fail to seek opinions from other qualified medical professionals or to acquire more specific knowledge on the different prostate cancer treatments. Instead, they agree to surgery and/or treatments they may not need or which have the risks of serious side effects.

But what if men discovered that there is a treatment available that is as effective as all other treatments and has few, if any, negative side effects?

Minimizing Risks of Treatment Side Effects

When I was told I had prostate cancer I was scared. Just the word cancer triggered fear. Like most men who are diagnosed with prostate cancer, I considered the surgery that was recommended to me by my urologist. After talking with a number of friends who had undergone surgery, I quickly discovered the high incidence of urinary incontinence, sexual dysfunction, and other unpleasant side effects associated with it.

As I looked at the available information on other prostate cancer treatments, I was overwhelmed by the amount of advertisements and websites claiming special expertise among their staff and implying that they were somehow the best place to go for prostate cancer treatment. After days of searching I discovered that many of the treatments on the most heavily marketed websites had significant adverse side effects. I was searching for a treatment with minimal side effects and eventually found one treatment that was different.

That treatment is proton therapy, a type of radiation therapy that is directed precisely to the cancer with minimal spread to healthy surrounding tissue. With this treatment most, if not all of the serious side effects so common in other treatments of prostate cancer, can be avoided. We are winning the war on cancer and in the forefront of this battle are the incredible successes associated with proton therapy.

Proton Warrior

This is my story about making my way through the perilous prostate cancer marketplace. It is directed to the one man in six who will get prostate cancer with the message that only one in 35 of us will actually die from it. It is a warning that not only must we be concerned about treating our cancer, we must be even more concerned about *how* we treat it.

I became a prostate cancer survivor by going through proton therapy at the MD Anderson Proton Therapy Center and not experiencing the bad side effects so common with other treatments. Based on my personal experience and observations as a patient, I not only saw the tremendous clinical effectiveness of proton therapy, I also discovered another powerful treatment component. Going through treatment as part of a strong, supportive social group of other patients, many of whom became my friends, was an unexpected bonus.

An interesting part of my journey involved going through prostate cancer treatment with a unique group of men that had said no to the treatment recommendation made by the urologist who diagnosed their prostate cancer. Instead of agreeing to their recommendations, sometimes made in a repeated and forceful manner, they looked elsewhere and sought additional information on the various ways to treat their prostate cancer. This behavior sets them apart from the vast majority of men who blindly go along with the recommendations made by their urologist. As these men studied the readily available information on the different ways of treating prostate cancer, they discovered that the most common types of treatment, surgery and, and to a lesser degree, conventional photon radiation, also have some of the most severe side effects. They did not want to experience these side effects and looked for a treatment that did not have them. By being able to say no to what their urologist recommended, they were able to avoid the sexual problems, urinary and fecal incontinence, and other side effects so common with other treatments. They went on to receive proton therapy, a treatment with significantly fewer side effects.

As I listened to the experiences other patients had with the urologist who diagnosed their prostate cancer and encountered more and more men who regretted going through surgery because of the serious side effects they were left with, something didn't seem right. In reviewing reports in the popular media and a cursory review of relevant research, I also discovered increasing criticism of the common treatments for prostate cancer. Most disheartening of all were the critical articles in some of our leading newspapers about how big money and big business have entered into the equation of how prostate cancer treatment is being provided,

I began to realize that something is amiss in the way we treat prostate cancer.

As I went through proton therapy treatment for my prostate cancer, I became an integral part of a support group of men who were also going through treatment with me. As we got to know each other and became friends, the analogy of combat came to my mind and with it the importance of how high morale and camaraderie among warriors contribute to their success in combat. When I joined the ranks of men fighting prostate cancer at the MD Anderson Proton

Therapy Center, I became one of the warriors in the battle against cancer.

Going through treatment and experiencing the positive effects of bonding with a number of my fellow patients, my confidence at beating prostate cancer grew. Gradually my thinking changed and I began to think of us as proton warriors. Needless to say, using the analogy of combat is a literary vehicle to explain how social support can enhance the effectiveness of an already effective treatment for prostate cancer. I was so impressed by the power of the social bonding I was experiencing, I had a banner made stating "Proton Warriors" and put it up in the patient changing area. I checked on it when I went for my one year check up and it was still there. It had many more signatures as new men signed it. If you go there, look for my name on this banner; it is on the lower right side. Then, go ahead and sign your name as well.

The Prostate Cancer Industry

My journey through prostate cancer treatment also led me to discover the "Prostate Cancer Industry," a growing part of the huge Medical Industrial Complex and a thriving billion dollar business based on marketing prostate cancer treatments. An increasing number of physicians are warning men diagnosed with prostate cancer not to rush into the treatment until they learn more about the side effects of the different treatments. Typical of such physicians is Dr. Bert Vorstman, a Florida based urologist who specializes in the use of high intensity focused ultrasound in the treatment of prostate cancer. He strongly encourages patients with localized prostate cancer to select treatment with minimal side effects. Dr. Vorstman recommends that patients and their spouses examine the various complications associated with each of the different treatment options for localized prostate cancer and determine how these different complications will impact their quality of life before selecting one. Dr. Vorstman states that incidence of these complications is profoundly different among the different treatments in that surgical options, including robotic removal, have the highest incidence of complications as well as the biggest negative impact on quality of life for both the man and his partner. Since the survival benefits among the major treatment groups for localized prostate cancer are similar whether the prostate has been surgically removed or not, he states patients with prostate cancer will be well advised to look at non-surgical options.[2]

I found myself wondering why, if the major treatments for prostate cancer are equally effective, so many men choose treatments with a high degree of risks for negative side effects. The answer to this question soon became apparent to me as more and more of the other patients going through treatment with me began to share their negative experiences of feeling pressured by the urologist who diagnosed their prostate cancer to accept treatment he/she recommended.

There is also the problem of overtreatment so effectively discussed in the book *Invasion of the Prostate Snatchers*[3] by cultural anthropologist Ralph Blum, who has held onto his cancerous prostate for the last 20 years, and Dr. Mark Scholz, a medical oncologist specializing in prostate cancer. One of the points they make is the overtreatment of prostate cancer that often leaves patients with serious side effects. Blum and Scholz state that studies have been published suggesting that over 75 percent of men diagnosed with prostate cancer are treated aggressively, even though most prostate cancers are slow-growing and will never pose a risk to their lives.

If, shortly after being diagnosed with prostate cancer, your urologist recommends a treatment he/she provides or refers you to an associate who provides the treatment, stand firm and tell him/her that you want time to review other options. Next, seek a second opinion from another physician unrelated to the first one. Also, turn to the Internet for help in identifying different prostate cancer treatments with minimal side effects.

If you want to minimize the adverse side effects common in treatment of prostate cancer you must acquire your own knowledge on prostate cancer so that you can make informed decisions. All you have to do is search the Internet for prostate cancer and you will discover a wealth of information. You will have to exercise some caution in reviewing this material, as some of it is misleading or inaccurate. Then, search proton therapy and you will see that this treatment is as effective as all other treatments but has the least side effects.

One of the problems with searching for information on prostate cancer on the web is finding accurate and complete information. There are a large number of sites put up by proponents of the various treatments for prostate cancer, manufacturers of the medical devices used to treat prostate cancer, and other segments of the medical industrial complex that are misleading. By doing your homework and obtaining as much information as you can from objective sources you are empowering yourself with knowledge of the different treatments and their side effects. One of the discoveries I made as I was going through proton therapy was that the overwhelming majority of patients going through treatment with me spent a considerable amount of time researching the various treatments for prostate cancer before deciding on their treatment. This is in contrast to the majority of men who are diagnosed with prostate cancer who simply follow the recommendations of their urologist. What happens is that they quickly agree to surgery or some form of conventional photon radiation, both of which have higher risks of side effects than proton therapy.

The reader who seeks accurate and complete information on the true side effects of the various prostate cancer treatments might feel severely challenged. For this reason men are encouraged to go to sites like the National Cancer Institute, American Cancer Society, as well as sites from centers that provide minimally invasive treatment such as proton therapy. The good news for men seeking proton therapy as a treatment for their prostate cancer is that an increasing number of proton therapy treatment centers are being built. The treatment machines are also getting smaller which will help to lower their costs. The result is that more and more men will have increased access to proton therapy treatment for their prostate cancer. It should be stated that at the time this book was published less than one percent of men with prostate cancer are being treated by proton therapy. Most men are receiving surgery and conventional photon radiation. The other fact to keep in mind is that not every man going through surgery or conventional photon radiation experience serious side effects. But enough of these men do experience serious side effects to raise caution and concern about selecting these treatments.

If, after you do your research and perhaps seek a second or even a third opinion and decide on proton therapy, your next step is in selecting a center that provides it. Information is provided in Appendix C on facilities that provide proton therapy. Once you get into proton therapy treatment you will discover the satisfaction of joining with your fellow patients in a tight, cohesive social group of men who were previously strangers when they first met but who quickly become friends. You will also be pleased with the ease of treatment and the almost total absence of any serious side effects.

I urge all of you reading this book that have recently been diagnosed with prostate cancer to consider proton therapy. Come join with those of us who have conquered prostate cancer and who have been largely spared from bad side effects so common with other treatments of prostate cancer. This is my story of conquering prostate cancer and avoiding adverse side effects. It can also become your story as you too can become a proton warrior. In the beginning of Blum and Scholz's excellent book *Invasion of the Prostate Snatchers*[3] Blum warns men "Prostate country is shadowy, misty territory, the Himalayas of masculine vulnerability. There are brigands lying in wait. And a shortage of reliable Sherpas." In his 2009 book *The Big Scare – The Business of Prostate Cancer*,[4] Urologist Anthony Horan points out the relative silence on unnecessary treatment and needless suffering men experience from the money generated from "The business of prostate cancer." My book joins the growing chorus of those warning about the dangers of either unnecessary treatment for prostate cancer or treatments with high risks of serious side effects not present in equally effective treatments. I urge those of you with localized prostate cancer with the tumor still encapsulated within the prostate to consider proton therapy. This book warns men newly diagnosed with prostate cancer that we must not only survive this cancer; we must also survive the perils the prostate cancer industry.

Chapter Two

Being Diagnosed with Prostate Cancer

"The day you find out is fine. But the next morning when you get up,
your knees are shaking. I didn't think I could make it to work."
Don Imus Discussing his diagnosis of prostate
cancer on his radio show, 3-16-09

Being Hit with the Unexpected

Years ago I read that one out of every four men will die from cancer. More recently I read that one of six men will be diagnosed with prostate cancer sometime during their life. Prior to acquiring this additional knowledge on prostate cancer, I was like many men in their 60's and beyond and even some younger including a surprising number of men in their 50's and even 40's who, when diagnosed with prostate cancer, knew little about it.

I was in my 40's when I first started having a digital rectal exam. At first, I had no idea why doctors were sticking their finger up my rectum in a procedure identified as a Digital Rectal Examination (DRE), but I quickly discovered that they were feeling my prostate. About the size of a walnut, the prostate straddles the urethral canal leading from the bladder to the tip of the penis and can be felt with a rubber gloved finger inserted into the rectum. I was also to discover later the key importance of the urethral canal when it comes to prostate cancer.

Up into my sixties the reassuring words of different doctors were "smooth and round," which meant no protrusions indicating the growth of cancer cells pushing against the wall of the prostate. Since every annual checkup always included blood work, I discovered the importance of one such test, the PSA or prostate specific antigen test. For many years my doctors would simply tell me everything was fine. I have never been overweight, kept physically active, was in good health and not on any medication. My only major surgery was having my right knee replaced resulting from rebuilding my home and business after they were destroyed by hurricane Katrina in 2005.

Prior to Katrina, my wife and I were living in a beautiful waterfront community in Pass Christian, Mississippi, a historical old town on the Mississippi Gulf Coast. When hurricane Katrina approached we fled to safety and stayed two weeks at a motel in Alabama. We then went to Springfield, MO to be near one of our two sons. When we returned a month later, we were appalled by the destruction we saw. We lost all of our records and belongings from our home and businesses that were flooded and damaged by the hurricane. What followed next was a yearlong ordeal of rebuilding our home and businesses. It was a period where the goodness in people became evident as many kind people rushed to provide aid and assistance. In my case, a number of Christian college students came and helped clean out a storage facility I owned.

After rebuilding post Katrina, life was good. I thought surviving Katrina would likely be my last difficult experience. I soon learned that another major challenge lay ahead.

"My Finger Tells Me Something's Not Right"

Around December of 2010, my new urologist was doing his digital exam when he exclaimed that he felt a slight bump on the right side of my prostate. Inserting his finger deeper in me and pressing it harder on the prostate he made the fateful statement "My finger tells me something is not right." Finishing his exam, he turned to me and stated he wanted to do a biopsy "just to make sure there was no cancer there."

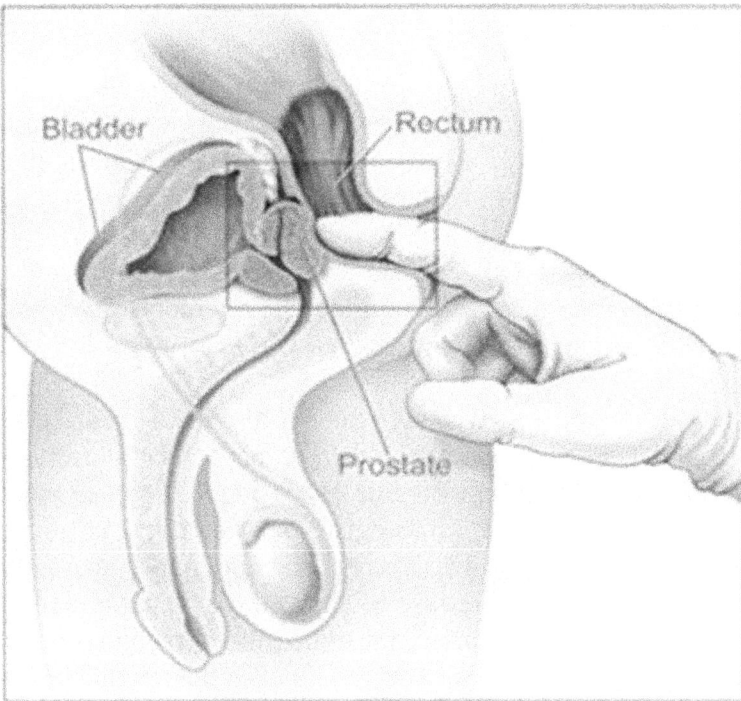

National Cancer Institute
General Information about Prostate Cancer

By the time men reach their 60's many of them have had a prostate biopsy. While it is not something one actively seeks for fun, it is not a particularly painful procedure. The doctor goes in through the rectum and to the side of the prostate. A mechanical device is used which punches into the prostate and withdraws a tissue sample. So, I was not overly concerned and had the biopsies. I am told that the typical number of biopsies is usually 12, sometimes more or less. I had 12 biopsies.

"You Have Prostate Cancer"

About 10 days later my doctor called me while I was enjoying a beer and watching the evening news.

"Mr. Dawley, this is Dr. Smith (a pseudonym), I'm calling to tell you that the biopsy results were positive."

Dr. Smith paused purposely, allowing the words to sink in.

"You have adenocancer, cancer of the prostate," he added and paused again as those words had the effect on me of suddenly being hit by a truck.

"But I don't want you to worry; your cancer is still very curable. You have a Gleason score of six and it is stage two," Dr. Smith added.

I was in a dream-like state hearing what he was saying and feeling adrift and outside of myself as he continued talking.

"My nurse will call you in the next week and set up an appointment to see me. It will be in the late afternoon and you will be my last patient. I will have all the time you want to go over this and discuss your options," Dr. Smith added.

Having worked for over 20 years in a general medical surgical hospital and having known a number of physicians personally, Dr. Smith was the most compassionate physician I had ever met. I felt fortunate having him as my urologist. He was a few years younger than me and presumably had earned enough money to retire if he wished but continued on because he enjoyed practicing urology

"In the meantime I want to run some more tests and my secretary will call you in a day or two when she makes the appointments," Dr. Smith concluded before we closed our discussion.

An appointment was set up later in the week for me to get a CAT scan and MRI not really understanding why these tests were being done.

Life Goes On

How am I going to tell Linda, my dear wife of 40 plus years, that I have cancer? I pondered back and forth as I awaited her return from one of the three dancing clubs to which she belongs.

I downed what was left of my beer and got another one. Time for some serious thinking, I mused to myself as I slowly drank my second beer.

By the time I had finished my third beer, I had a plan. I decided to play it cool and would nonchalantly mention to Linda that I have a mild case of prostate cancer. A third beer had relaxed me somewhat and made me think I could get her to take the news in stride.

"Hello, I'm home…" I heard the cheerful voice of Linda as she came in through our garage after dancing at a community event with one of her dance clubs.

"How did it go?" I asked smiling broadly.

I listened carefully and attentively (not my usual style) as she excitedly described her dance events.

With my heart rate slightly up and straining to keep my cool, I casually mentioned that Dr. Smith had called and I have a mild case of prostate cancer.

It was like a rifle shot being fired in terms of the startled reaction it generated in Linda.

"WHAT DID YOU SAY!!!"

"Now calm down honey. The biopsy results were positive for prostate cancer but he tells me we caught it early and I have a very good chance of having it cured."

Tears welled up in Linda's eyes as she sat on our living room sofa looking at me with terror etched on her face.

For the next hour Linda and I discussed what Dr. Smith had told me. I sometimes don't attend to details when someone tells me something, plus, when I heard the word cancer I got scared and then heard even less. Linda is a detail person and wants to know every single aspect of whatever catches her attention. "The bottom line (one of my favorite expressions next to 'the big picture') is that the prognosis for me is very good," I told Linda. I kept trying to get her to relax and to look at the positive information Dr. Smith had given me about my cancer. Linda finally settled down but I could tell she was still scared.

I am an optimist and always look on the bright side. After the terror of being told I had cancer subsided a bit, I found myself thinking how lucky I was to have lived such a good life. I have a wonderful wife and two great sons plus two lovely daughters-in-law and a precious grandson and two delightful granddaughters. Over the years of working with people who were dealing with serious health problems, I learned that it helps to think of what is the worst that could happen and then try to accept that. In my case, I had lived a full and productive life. I assumed that I would live at least three years more if I had the worst type of cancer and if that was all I had left, I was going to make the most of it. Soon, I was able to come to terms with having prostate cancer.

It was more difficult for Linda and she was obviously controlling herself. She was careful not to cry or break down anymore. She was trying to be strong for my sake and I loved her even more for doing so. But that evening her soft sobbing woke me up at four AM. Rolling over to her I held her in my arms and softly told her everything would be okay even though I had some self-doubt.

My Treatment Options

Linda and I met with Dr. Smith five days after his call telling me I had prostate cancer. He began by telling me that the MRI and CAT scan did not show any progression or spreading of the cancer outside of my prostate. He indicated that this finding was important and that it would be easier to treat as a result. Linda had a large number of questions and Dr. Smith patiently answered all of them. I listened carefully to everything said. "You are healthy, not on any medication don't have heart disease, hypertension, or diabetes so the option of "Watchful Waiting" would not be appropriate for you", Dr. Smith told me softly adding "the chances are that prostate cancer would eventually kill you if you don't seek active treatment."

Dr. Smith stated that watchful waiting is appropriate for many older men who are not in good health because of the odds of their dying from something else being greater than their dying from prostate cancer.

Dr. Smith then summarized the treatment options. He began by stating that all of them worked and all had side effects. He first discussed radiation in which my prostate and surrounding area would be radiated and added that the negative side effects would be radiation burns on the urethra and rectum which could lead to urinary and fecal incontinence and erectile dysfunction. Next he discussed the use of radioactive seeds being implanted in my prostate. This also had side effects. He felt this was not a treatment for me. He then described surgery, radical prostatectomy, or the total removal of the prostate using a new procedure called robotic surgery. While he added that there were some possible side effects, he felt this was the best treatment for me. He continued on for an additional twenty minutes or so carefully answering our questions. He concluded by urging me to do my own research and seek additional opinions because of the importance of my making the best decision.

"The Best Surgeon in Town"

I asked Dr. Smith again about what he recommended, and he described the relatively new procedure of robotic surgery in which a small camera and other tools are inserted through small holes in the abdomen and the prostate is then removed. He then described the skill of his new partner, a younger man who had acquired skill in doing the robotic prostatectomy. He did NOT use the term I was to hear so often from my fellow prostate cancer patients who stated their doctor described the person who they recommended to do the surgery as being "the best surgeon in town." Dr. Smith nonetheless impressed me so much that I believed (and still believe) that his partner is indeed skilled at this procedure.

Thanking Dr. Smith, Linda and I left feeling somewhat better. I was leaning toward having his partner do the radical prostatectomy. Before finalizing my decision, I followed his advice and decided to do some more research.

Scared and Vulnerable

Men are all alike in that after being diagnosed with prostate cancer we experience fear and uncertainty. It is a period in which we are quite vulnerable as we have the need for someone to step up and tell us what is best for us in terms of treatment. This fear comes from not knowing much about prostate cancer and the normal natural desire of not wanting to be killed by it. My urologist apparently knew from experience that this is a difficult period and that most men need more time and knowledge before deciding on a treatment so that they can make an informed decision. His insistence that I do research and seek a second opinion impressed me and I did just that. But, in the meantime, life goes on.

Our New Year's Eve Party

After you are diagnosed with prostate cancer there will likely be a period of time in which your life more or less continues as it had previously. This a crucial period and while it may not be evident to us it is a time when our mind churns through all of the information we have acquired as we slowly decide on what we want to do about our prostate cancer. For me, this period occurred during our involvement in our 2011 New Year's Eve party.

Prior to my learning I had prostate cancer we had planned a New Year's Eve party at our home. We are fortunate in having a large number of friends and went about sending out our invitations. To our pleasant surprise almost everyone was able to come. Our minds focused on the upcoming party and we were able to forget the cancer growing in my prostate.

For the next five days Linda lost herself in the fun of decorating our garage and house for the party. She hung streamers across the ceiling, installed Christmas lights, and placed a white material over all of my tools and workbench hiding them from view. She also downloaded Golden Oldies dance music and planned some games. We got some good news when two of our friends asked if they could bring the Episcopalian priest of our church and his lovely wife to our party.

The party was a great success and everyone had fun.

I only told two of our guests that I had prostate cancer, my best friend and fellow psychologist Sal Guidry and his wife Brynn. That evening Linda and I were both feeling the warmth of good friends and were moved to express the pleasure we felt at having our friends join us for the evening.

Standing before everyone, I got their attention and stated: "I just want to let you know how pleased Linda and I are for all of you to be here tonight sharing this evening with us," I started out.

As I looked around I could see that my emotion was being met with similar emotions.

"As Linda and I grow older we realize more than ever how important friends are to us. And since you are our dear friends, enjoying this evening with you makes us very happy. We want to thank all of you for coming."

Linda then stated that she too appreciated everyone coming and spending the evening with us and it was a very special event for her.

Applause followed as I made my way back for another glass of red wine.

I don't want to glorify excessive consumption of alcohol or to give the impression of being an alcoholic. I seldom drink more than three alcoholic drinks on any occasion. I discuss the drinking I did that night to let you know that night was different for me. After all, I was now a cancer patient, plus, for some strange inexplicable reason, I felt positive about my treatment. This feeling in turn led to a greater degree of appreciation for the good life I've lived and brought me back for another glass of wine.

At midnight, I opened the double door of the garage and we all went outside to the pleasant 70 degrees Gulf Coast night. It was kissing time as all the men kissed all of the women. Then, as a former Marine Corps bugler, it was time for me to present the neighborhood with a melody of Marine Corps bugle calls. With a good lip and red wine confidence I played reveille, pay call, chow call, and charge, on which I stumbled a bit.

As our friends left each stated that they had a wonderful time and thanked us for inviting them.

That night, Linda and I slept well. Tucked in our bed we were comforted by the warmth of our having close friends. Instead of arising at my usual 5 AM, I slept until 10:45 AM. I awoke with a slight hangover but still felt great.

I was now ready to face my next task on the road to conquering prostate cancer.

You have or will likely experience something similar during the crucial time frame between being diagnosed with prostate cancer and selecting what you believe to be the best treatment for you. This will be one of the most life altering decisions you will need to make. It is crucial that you fully understand your prostate cancer. The next chapter is my effort to provide much of the information you need to know. It may be a bit dry and technical, but once you master it you will be better equipped to continue your journey.

Chapter Three

Understanding Your Prostate Cancer

"The words "it's cancer," when spoken to you by a doctor, are among the most distressing in the language. To say that hearing them leaves you reeling would not be overstating it. And yet oddly, of all possible cancers, cancer of the prostate would be my cancer of choice."[1]

Ralph Blum, *Invasion of the Prostate Snatchers*

Learning About Your Enemy

For those of us who are newly diagnosed with prostate cancer it is the beginning of a learning process as we try to understand the enemy attacking us. A few men do research comparable to a doctoral dissertation while most barely scratch the surface and blindly agree to what their physician recommends. But what we all have in common is that once we are diagnosed with prostate cancer we all want to know just how bad is the condition. Since prostate cancer is so common, many of us have friends and relatives who have been treated for it and they are a valuable source of information. As we start gathering information on prostate cancer we quickly discover that in most instances it is a slow growing cancer and treatment success is high. At this point we breathe a sigh of relief. After a pause, we then begin to look more closely at the side effects of the various treatments and this is where serious research pays off. This chapter is intended to give you the basics of understanding your prostate cancer. It will cover key factors crucial to your cancer and the type of treatment you may receive and includes such matters as your Gleason score, your Stage, and the role of the PSA score. Chapter Four, will cover the various treatment options.

Understanding Prostate Cancer and Ways to Treat It

Prostate Gland: The prostate is a gland the size of a walnut located beneath the bladder and surrounds the urethra just below the bladder and is part of the male reproductive system. The prostate gland can be felt during a digital rectal exam discussed later.

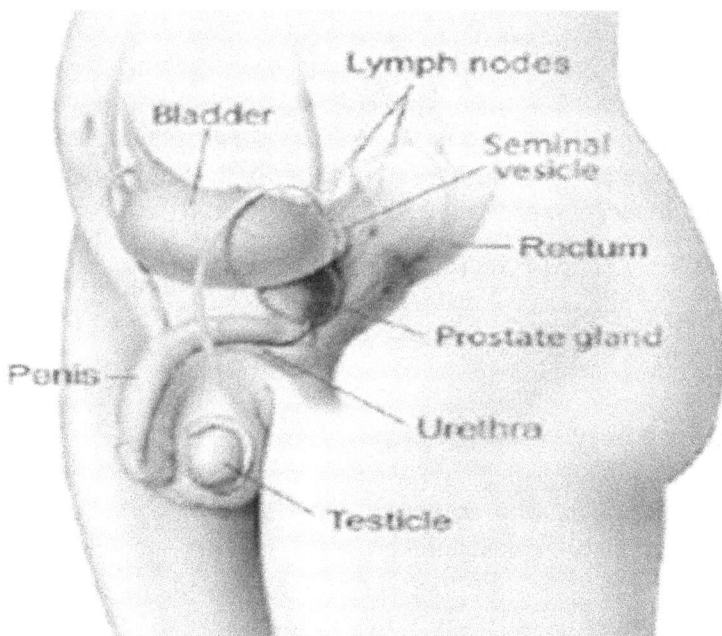

National Cancer Institute
About Prostate Cancer

The prostate is a gland that helps make semen. Semen is the milky fluid that carries sperm from the testicles through the penis during ejaculation. The prostate is part of the male reproductive system. It has sections, which are called lobes. The prostate lies low in the pelvis, below the bladder and in front of the rectum and surrounds part of the urethra, the tube that carries urine out of the bladder and through the penis.

Prostate Cancer

When cancer occurs in the prostate it is identified as prostate cancer. While most prostate cancer is slow growing, a small percentage of cases is fast growing cancer and it is for this reason that as men we need to have regular checkups. In aggressive prostate cancer there is the danger it may metastasize and spread to other parts of the body especially to the bones and lymph nodes. Prostate cancer generally occurs in older men over fifty and when diagnosed it is slow growing in about 3/4 of the cases with 1/4 of cases being fast growing. Many men die from other causes of death even though upon autopsy are found to have prostate cancer. Depending on the type of cancer, various treatment options are available.

Key Treatment Variables

Your Gleason Score

The single most important laboratory report you will receive is the determination of the structure of the cancer cells removed in the biopsy. Typically three different pathologists study these cells under a microscope and rank them based on their cell structure. A number of biopsies are performed ranging usually from nine to 12. Slides are prepared and three different pathologists do independent scoring of the structure of the cells to determine the aggressiveness of your cancer. The pathologist studies the cell structure to determine its variation from normal cell structure. There are five categories reflecting the degree of differentiation of the cancerous cell structure from the structure of a normal cell. If your cancer cells look like a normal cell they are called well-differentiated cells. If they differ significantly from normal cells they are called poorly differentiated. The more poorly differentiated your cancer cells are, the more aggressive is your cancer. The pathologists will assign a score of from one to five to indicate the degree of the most common cell structure. The pathologist then studies the next most common cell structure and assigns another score from one to five. The resultant scores are then added together and represent your Gleason score. The most commonly found scores are 5, 6, and 7. Scores of 8,9, and10 reflect faster growing cancers. Scores of 4 and below are rare and represent slow growing cancer and often do not necessitate immediate treatment.

Prostate Specific Antigen Test (PSA)

The Prostate Specific Antigen or PSA is an enzyme your body uses to turn semen that has congealed after an ejaculation back into a liquid and is a widely used measurement in diagnosing prostate cancer. Even though the PSA is used as a screening tool and does have limitations, it remains as one of the most widely used indicators of prostate cancer. Critics of using the PSA to diagnose cancer point out that other factors can also increase the PSA such as prostatitis, recent ejaculation either by intercourse or masturbation, the presence of benign prostatic hyperplasia or enlarged prostate or simply by engaging in physical activity such as riding a bike before the blood sample was drawn. A repeat blood sample is typically taken when a high PSA is found just in case it was artificially elevated by something other than cancer. Both a high PSA, generally over 4 and a rapidly rising PSA can indicate prostate cancer.

There is some evidence indicating the clinical usefulness of a variant of the PSA blood test called free PSA. It has been found that men who have prostate cancer compared to men who have an enlarged prostate referred to as benign prostatic hypertrophy have lower percentage of free PAS in their blood. There is growing consensus for the value of measuring free PSA in diagnosing prostate cancer, particularly for men in whom total PSA is between 4 and 10 and who have a negative digital rectal exam or DRE. There is also a growing controversy over the use of the PSA for screening otherwise healthy men for the risks of prostate cancer. This issue will be discussed in more detail later in this book.

Staging

Staging refers to the size and extent of the prostate cancer and is the process your physician uses to determine its advancement and aggressiveness. Early stage prostate cancer that is localized to the prostate and has not spread outside it is described as stages I and II. When cancer has spread beyond the prostate to the seminal vessels, it is described as Stage III and is frequently referred to as locally advanced disease. Stage IV is when the cancer has spread beyond the seminal vesicles to lymph nodes and/or to other tissues or organs.

The American Joint Committee on Cancer (AJCC) is the most widely used staging system and uses the TNM System and is summarized below.

The TNM System:

1. T category – a rating of the extent of the primary tumor
2. N category – a rating of the spread of the tumor and whether or not it has spread to nearby lymph nodes
3. M category – The most important variable as it establishes the absence or presence of distant metastasis

All three of the above categories are used together to the overall stage of your cancer.

T categories (clinical)

There are 4 categories for describing the local extent of the prostate tumor, ranging from T1 to T4. Most of these have subcategories as well.

T1: Your doctor can't feel the tumor or see it with imaging such as transrectal ultrasound.

T1a: The cancer is found incidentally (by accident) during a transurethral resection of the prostate (often abbreviated as TURP) that was done for benign prostatic hyperplasia (BPH). Cancer is present in less than 5% of the tissue removed.

T1b: The cancer is found during a TURP but is present in more than 5% of the tissue removed.

T1c: The cancer is found by needle biopsy that was done because of an increased PSA.

T2: Your doctor can feel the cancer when a digital rectal exam (DRE) is done, but it still appears to be confined to the prostate gland.

T2a: The cancer is in one half or less of only one side (left or right) of your prostate.

T2b: The cancer is in more than half of only one side (left or right) of your prostate.

T2c: The cancer is in both sides of your prostate.

T3: The cancer has begun to grow and spread outside your prostate and may involve the seminal vesicles.

T3a: The cancer extends outside the prostate but not to the seminal vesicles.

T3b: The cancer has spread to the seminal vesicles.

T4: The cancer has grown into tissues next to your prostate (other than the seminal vesicles), such as the urethral sphincter (muscle that helps control urination), the rectum, and/or the wall of the pelvis.

N categories

N0: The cancer has not spread to any lymph nodes.

N1: The cancer has spread to one or more regional (nearby) lymph nodes in the pelvis.

M categories

M0: The cancer has not spread beyond the regional lymph nodes.

M1: The cancer has spread beyond the regional nodes.

M1a: The cancer has spread to distant (outside of the pelvis) lymph nodes.

M1b: The cancer has spread to the bones.

M1c: The cancer has spread to other organs such as lungs, liver, or brain (with or without spread to the bones).

Stage Groupings – How Advanced is Your Prostate Cancer?

Once the T, N, and M categories have been determined, this information is combined, along with the Gleason score and PSA, in a process called stage grouping. If the Gleason score or PSA results are not available, the stage can be based on the T, N, and M categories. The overall stage is expressed in Roman numerals from I (the least advanced) to IV (the most advanced). This is done to help determine treatment options and the treatment prognosis.

Stage I: One of the Following Applies:

T1, N0, M0, Gleason score 6 or less, PSA less than 10: The doctor can't feel the tumor or see it with imaging such as transrectal ultrasound (it was either found during a transurethral resection or was diagnosed by needle biopsy done for a high PSA) [T1]. The cancer is still within the prostate and has not spread to lymph nodes [N0] or elsewhere in the body [M0]. The Gleason score is 6 or less and the PSA level is less than 10. OR

T2a, N0, M0, Gleason score 6 or less, PSA less than 10: The tumor can be felt on digital rectal exam or seen on transrectal ultrasound and is in one half or less of only one side (left or right) of your prostate [T2a]. The cancer is still within the prostate and has not spread to lymph nodes [N0] or elsewhere in the body [M0]. The Gleason score is 6 or less and the PSA level is less than 10.

Stage IIA: One of the Following Applies:

T1, N0, M0, Gleason score of 7, PSA less than 20: The doctor can't feel the tumor or see it with imaging such as transrectal ultrasound (it was either found during a transurethral resection or was diagnosed by needle biopsy done for a high PSA level) [T1]. The cancer has not spread to nearby lymph nodes [N0] or elsewhere in the body [M0].The tumor has a Gleason score of 7. The PSA level is less than 20. OR

T1, N0, M0, Gleason score of 6 or less, PSA at least 10 but less than 20: The doctor can't feel the tumor or see it with imaging such as transrectal ultrasound (it was either found during a transurethral resection or was diagnosed by needle biopsy done for a high PSA [T1]. The cancer has not spread to nearby lymph nodes [N0] or elsewhere in the body [M0]. The tumor has a Gleason score of 6 or less. The PSA level is at least 10 but less than 20. OR

T2a or T2b, N0, M0, Gleason score of 7 or less, PSA less than 20: The tumor can be felt on digital rectal exam or seen on transrectal ultrasound and is in only one side of the prostate [T2a or T2b]. The cancer has not spread to nearby lymph nodes [N0] or elsewhere in the body [M0]. It has a Gleason score of 7 or less. The PSA level is less than 20.

Stage IIB: One of the Following Applies:

T2c, N0, M0, any Gleason score, any PSA: The tumor can be felt on digital rectal exam or seen on transrectal ultrasound and is in both sides of the prostate [T2c]. The cancer has not spread to nearby lymph nodes [N0] or elsewhere in the body [M0]. The tumor can have any Gleason score and the PSA can be any value. OR

T1 or T2, N0, M0, any Gleason score, PSA of 20 or more: The cancer has not yet begun to spread outside the prostate. It may (or may not) be felt by digital rectal exam or seen on transrectal ultrasound [T1 or T2] The cancer has not spread to nearby lymph nodes [N0] or elsewhere in the body [M0]. The tumor can have any Gleason score. The PSA level is at least 20. OR

T1 or T2, N0, M0, Gleason score of 8 or higher, any PSA: The cancer has not yet begun to spread outside the prostate. It may (or may not) be felt by digital rectal exam or seen on transrectal ultrasound [T1 or T2]. The cancer has not spread to nearby lymph nodes [N0] or elsewhere in the body [M0]. The Gleason score is 8 or higher. The PSA can be any value.

Stage III:

T3, N0, M0, any Gleason score, any PSA: The cancer has begun to spread outside the prostate and may have spread to the seminal vesicles [T3], but it has not spread to the lymph nodes [N0] or elsewhere in the body [M0]. The tumor can have any Gleason score and the PSA can be any value.

Stage IV: One of the Following Applies:

T4, N0, M0, any Gleason score, any PSA: The cancer has spread to tissues next to the prostate (other than the seminal vesicles), such as the urethral sphincter (muscle that helps control urination), rectum, and/or the wall of the pelvis [T4]. The cancer has not spread to nearby lymph nodes [N0] or elsewhere in the body [M0]. The tumor can have any Gleason score and the PSA can be any value. OR

Any T, N1, M0, any Gleason score, any PSA: The tumor may be growing into tissues near the prostate [any T]. The cancer has spread to the lymph nodes (N1) but has not spread elsewhere in the body [M0]. The tumor can have any Gleason score and the PSA can be any value. OR

Any T, any N, M1, any Gleason score, any PSA: The cancer may be growing into tissues near the prostate [any T] and may have spread to nearby lymph nodes [any N]. It has spread to other, more distant sites in the body [M1]. The tumor can have any Gleason score and the PSA can be any value.

Other Staging Systems

In addition to the TNM system, other systems have been used to stage prostate cancer. The Whitmore-Jewett system, which stages prostate cancer as A, B, C, or D, was commonly used in the past, but most prostate specialists now use the TNM system. If your doctors use the Whitmore-Jewett system, ask them to translate it into the TNM system or to explain how their staging will determine your treatment options.

Chapter Four

Types of Prostate Cancer Treatments and their Side Effects

Select your prostate cancer treatment in haste and
repent at your leisure.

Selecting a Treatment

Provided next are reviews of available treatments for prostate cancer with attention focused on the two treatments 90% + of men receive: surgery and conventional photon radiation. These two treatments are then compared with the treatment I received, proton therapy. While the following information will be helpful, you are urged to also read information from other sources. To become fully informed you need to study surgery, both robotic and non-robotic surgery, as well as material from those who advocate conventional photon radiation. There are also those who advocate Intensity Modulated Radiation Therapy (IMRT), Brachytherapy and other treatments such as High Intensity Focused Ultrasound (HIFU). You are also advised to consult with different health care facilities offering the different treatments options so that you can better understand the pros and cons of each treatment. It is very important to obtain information on the risk of side effects before selecting a treatment.

The Different Treatments for Prostate Cancer

For many of us, being diagnosed with prostate cancer can lead to a confusing, fear-laden period as we try to figure how we want to proceed. Many men will listen to their urologist and follow his or her recommendations for treatment. With a huge amount of information easily available on the Internet, doing research on different treatments for prostate cancer is now very easy and increasing numbers of men are doing so. As you search you will soon discover the large amount of information put out by proponents of the different treatments. Reviewing this information can be confusing as it is often incomplete and misleading. Side effects of the treatment each website is promoting are downplayed. Many sites will include proton therapy and conventional photon radiation together and identify them both as radiation treatment. Categorizing these two different treatments that way leads to confusion, in that proton therapy has significantly fewer side effects than conventional photon radiation.

There are natural biases that come into play among different medical specialties with surgeons tending to recommend surgery and radiologists tending to recommend radiation. It is thus advantageous for newly diagnosed men to seek second or third opinions from other medical specialists such as their family physician or internist or a medical oncologist. In this section the two most common types of treatment for prostate cancer, surgery and conventional photon radiation, are discussed followed by a discussion of proton therapy.

Here are your options once you have been diagnosed with prostate cancer.

Watchful Waiting Verses Active Treatment

Ralph Blum has lived with prostate cancer for over twenty years. He attributes his survival to having "Low Risk" rather than "Aggressive" prostate cancer. Working closely with his medical oncologist Dr. Mark Scholz, Blum has avoided active treatment and the side effects associated with it. He has become what he refers to as a "refusenik" by not entering into active treatment and states "The track I have followed has been scary at times, a cross between a high wire walk and a military exercise with live ammunition."[1] He has no regrets about the path he elected to follow. About 80% of prostate cancers are candidates for watchful waiting in that their prostate cancer is also low risk. Being followed by a medical oncologist or other medical specialists is a key part of watchful waiting.

Once you've been diagnosed with prostate cancer, there are two options, temporarily forgo treatment and wait and see what happens (watchful waiting) or seek active treatment. Since some types of prostate cancer pose little immediate threat such as Stage I and some Stage II cancers with a Gleason score below 6, prompt treatment is not always indicated. Furthermore, if a recently diagnosed man is old and in relatively poor health, the chances are that he will die from something other than prostate cancer. In both cases watchful waiting may be recommended.

In watchful waiting your physician will follow you closely and monitor your tumor with DRE every six to 12 months plus checks of your PSA during these time frames. Your physician will also look closely for any physical symptoms such as painful urination, increased difficulty controlling your urine, increased nighttime urination and increased sexual problems. Whenever any signs occur suggesting the possibility of prostate cancer growing at a faster rate, another biopsy will be done. If more advanced cancer is detected, your physician will then recommend one or more of the following treatments.

Different Types of Active Treatment

The established types of active treatments available for prostate cancer are listed below:
1. Surgery
2. Conventional Photon Radiation Therapy
3. Proton Radiation Therapy
4. Hormone Therapy
5. Chemotherapy
6. High-Intensity Focused Ultrasound (not yet approved in the USA)
7. Cryosurgery
8. Other treatments

Selecting a treatment depends on several factors such as your age, the aggressiveness of your cancer based on your Gleason score, and the number of tissue samples from the biopsy that contain cancer cells. Other important factors include the stage of the cancer, the symptoms being experienced, your general health and age.

All Major Prostate Cancer Treatments Are Equally Effective but Differ Significantly in their Side Effects

The consensus in the medical field is that all of the widely used treatments including proton therapy work equally well in terms of treating prostate cancer. The real differentiating factor for these treatments is the degree of negative side effects commonly associated with each of them. And this is where the picture becomes confusing. Much of the literature put out by proponents of different treatments downplay any side effects associated with the treatment they are promoting. There is a great deal of misinformation on the Internet and getting more accurate information about the side effects of various treatments can be difficult. The treatments will be discussed in three main categories: Surgery, Radiation, and Other Treatments. Because of the importance of side effects, a large part of this Chapter is devoted to discussing them.

Surgery

"Out of 50,000 radical prostatectomy's performed every year in the United States alone, more than 40,000 are unnecessary. In other words, the vast majority of men with prostate cancer would have lived just as long without any operation at all. Most did not need to have their sexuality cut out". [1]

Mark Scholz, M.D.
Invasion of the Prostate Snatchers

Surgery is usually done on men with early (Stage I or II) prostate cancer. It's sometimes done on men with Stage III or IV prostate cancer. The surgeon may remove the whole prostate or only part of it. Before the surgeon removes the prostate, the lymph nodes in the pelvis may be removed. If prostate cancer cells are found in the lymph nodes, the disease may have spread to other parts of the body and the surgeon may not remove the prostate and instead may suggest other types of treatment. Whenever surgery of any type is done and the prostate is removed, it is referred to as "radical prostatectomy. This surgical procedure involves removing the prostate, surrounding tissue, and seminal vessels. The bladder is then pulled down in the void left by the removed prostate and the surgeon then resections the part of the urethra from the bladder that has been pulled down to the remaining part of the urethra left after the removal of the prostate.

There are several types of surgery for prostate cancer. Each type has significant risks.

Types of Surgery

Open Prostatectomy

Open Prostatectomy is also called retropubic prostatectomy. In this surgery, your doctor removes the prostate through a single long cut made in your abdomen from a point below your navel to just above the pubic bone. He or she might also check nearby lymph nodes for cancer (see drawing below). This type of surgery can be used for nerve sparing. Nerve-sparing surgery lessens the chances that the nerves near your prostate will be harmed. These important nerves control erections and normal bladder function.

Laparoscopic Surgery

In this type of surgery, your doctor uses a laparoscope to see and remove the prostate. A laparoscope is a long slender tube with a light and camera on the end. This surgery is done through 4 to 6 small cuts in the navel and the abdomen, instead of a single long cut in the abdomen. The laparoscope is inserted through one of the cuts, and surgery tools are inserted through the others. A robot can be used to do this type of surgery. This type of surgery can also be used for nerve-sparing surgery.

Perineal Prostatectomy.

In this type of surgery, your doctor removes the prostate through an incision between your scrotum and anus. With this method, the surgeon is not able to check the lymph nodes for cancer and nerve-sparing surgery is more difficult to do. This type of surgery is not used very often.

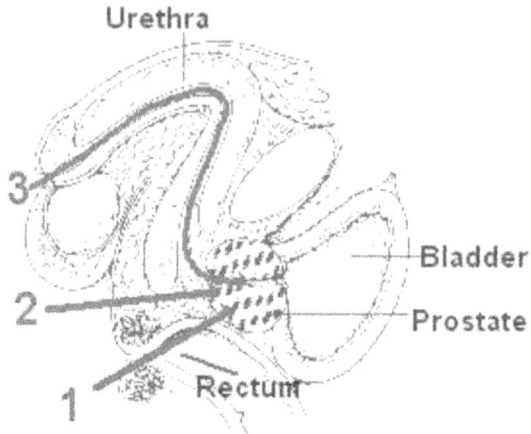

Approaches to the prostate
Transrectal approach
Transperineal approach
Transurethral resection

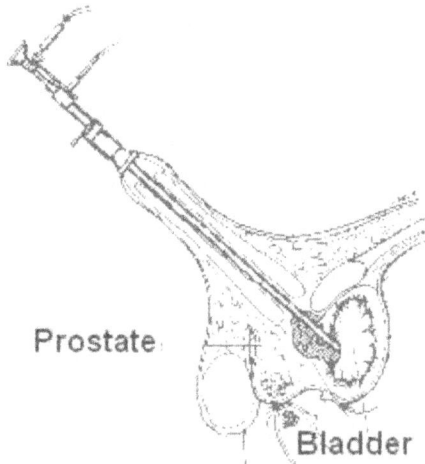

Transurethral resection

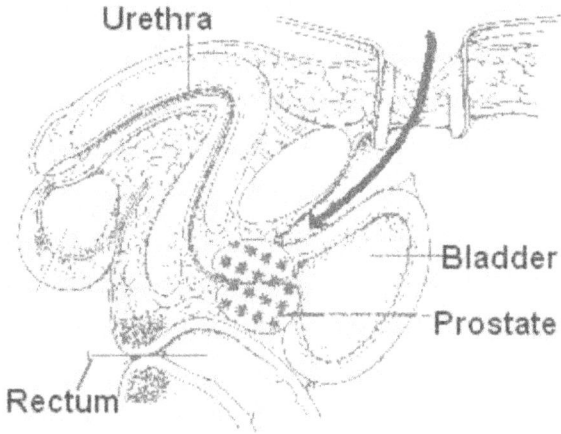

Retropubic prostatectomy
National Cancer Institute

Robotic Surgery

This is a relatively new technique whose proponents point out as being quicker with less down time. This procedure still may result in serious side effects. It evolved from efforts by the military to allow surgeons to operate via the internet/television on wounded personnel far away on distant battlefields. In this procedure a number of small openings are made in the abdomen into which a small television camera and surgical implements are inserted. A small incision from 5 mm-12 mm in length is made only requiring 4 to 6 small incisions. These incisions allow instruments to pass through ports (a hollow cylinder through which instruments can pass), keeping the surgeon's hands outside the patient. The surgeon does not use his hands in this procedure but instead sits 5 to 10 feet or so away remotely operating implements that allow him to surgically remove the prostate. He sits at a console where he views a computer monitor while using a joy stick to carry out the surgical procedure.

Is Robotic Surgery Better than Open Surgery?

The use of robotic surgery has grown significantly going from around one percent of prostate cancer surgeries in 2003 to 80% of all prostate cancer surgeries in 2011. The rate of robotic surgery is even higher now as more and more hospitals, clinics, and groups of urologists are purchasing one of the devices. The National Cancer Institute Cancer Bulletin reported on a study by Dr. Jim C. Hu of Brigham and Women's Hospital in Boston, which found that men who underwent robotic surgery had twice the risk of genitourinary complication, a 30 percent increased risk, and a 40 percent increased risk of erectile dysfunction 18 months after the procedure compared with men who underwent the conventional open prostate cancer surgery. Given the available data on standard open surgery compared to robotic surgery, Rabin quotes Dr. Hu as stating that open surgery should remain the "gold standard" for men who opt for surgery to treat localized prostate cancer."[2]

Urologist Dr. Bert Vorstman criticizes all types of surgical removal of the prostate in treating prostate cancer. Vorstman states that robotic surgery has become so entrenched in the mindset of many treating physicians that "...they have given it the arbitrary moniker of being the 'gold standard." Vorstman states there is no justification for calling surgery the "gold standard" for treating prostate cancer. He goes on to state that when this term is "recited enough some surgeons actually believe it." Vorstman further states that although the complications of impotence and incontinence are so common after surgery that they are seen by surgeons "as the cost of doing business" yet are "often dismissed (with feigned surprise) by the treating surgeon as unusual." Vorstman is critical of the clever marketing efforts sponsored to a large extent by the manufacturers of robotic surgery devices. He states "Another marketing spin is using the term 'minimally invasive' to advertise this surgery. There is nothing minimally invasive about this 'high tech robotic procedure as removal of the prostate still requires hospitalization."[3]

Increasing numbers of urologists are now performing robotic surgery for prostate cancer. It seems like every medical center is now providing this procedure even though the available evidence seems to suggest that it leaves patients with more severe side effects than the conventional open surgery, which has its share of serious side effects.

Are There Any Advantages of Surgery?

The actual surgery is generally a quick procedure in which some men can go in a hospital, have the surgery that day, and, if there are no serious complications, are discharged two or three days later. All will wear a catheter for a week or so and have some minor discomfort. While surgery is relatively quick, recovery from it can still last up to 12 weeks. Depending on the degree of the side effects, life can, to a certain extent, go on as usual in the sense of being able to return to work and engage in most regular activities during recovery. The problem is that according to many studies there is a significant risk of experiencing serious side effects such as incontinence or impotence and other problems following surgery.

What to Keep in Mind When Considering Surgery

Is Surgery Justified?

The overriding question in regard to surgery is whether or not it is justified. This is a determination all men diagnosed with prostate cancer will need to make in consultation with several types of medical specialists including medical oncologists. In those instances in which treatment is indicated, the pros and cons of surgery are discussed next.

Prostate Surgery Can Be Difficult:

It is widely acknowledged that when it comes to surgery, the skill of the surgeon is of crucial importance. If you are considering surgery you need to keep in mind that the surgical removal of the prostate is a tedious, difficult operation and the success of the procedure and likelihood of side effects hinge on the skill of the surgeon.

Even the Most Skilled Surgeons Sometimes Don't Do Well:

For many years the record holder for the greatest number of home runs being hit in baseball was Babe Ruth. What many people don't realize is that Ruth also held another record, that of having the greatest number of strikeouts. The field of sports is filled with remarkably talented players who have one thing in common – their high level of skill. But as anyone familiar with sports knows the level of skill in star athletes can vary from time to time and may be influenced by such factors as how rested is he or she, something on his/her mind that may be distracting him/her, or any other number of factors. Even athletes with the greatest degree of skill don't always hit home runs or throw the winning pass for a touchdown. Instead, they sometimes fumble, throw an interception, or strike out. No one can be perfect all of the time. Just as no skilled athlete scores every time they play, no surgeon is perfect every time he or she operates. That's just the nature of skill. There is a normally occurring variation among human beings when they perform a task going from performing some skill very well to doing it less well, to sometimes doing it not well at all, and finally to sometimes just plain doing it badly. It is for this reason that surgeons pay such huge amounts of money for malpractice insurance and why there is a whole industry built around medical malpractice.

Some Surgeons Are Less Skilled:

In 2010 I and just about every other fan of the New Orleans Saints football team were glued to TV screen every time they played. That year something incredible happened; the New Orleans Saints won the Super Bowl. While the team as a whole played superbly throughout the season, there were some team members who did not live up to their expectations. Even though they were paid very well and were clearly motivated to play well, they just couldn't deliver. It's the same in medicine and every other profession. There are some people in certain jobs that do not perform well. In virtually every work setting one can find people who are not good at what they are doing. Why should the field of surgery be any different from teaching, engineering, or automobile mechanics? The reality is that there are physicians that are not good at what they are doing. So, for anyone determined to have prostate cancer surgery or any type of difficult surgery they would be well advised to seek out a good surgeon. Doing so is, unfortunately, not easy. Even if a good surgeon is used, there is still no guarantee of a successful outcome in terms of minimal side effects.

Are You Willing To Chance It?

How can you make sure you find a skilled surgeon? The answer is that there really are not any good ways to know who is good and, more importantly, who is not good. There is reluctance among physicians to criticize each other and while those same physicians make sure to steer their loved ones and friends away from other physicians who are not good, the average patient considering surgery does not always have access to such information. So, finding a surgeon who is skilled is a big factor. Another thought to keep in mind when considering surgery is that even the best surgeon is only human and is thus liable to making mistakes and having an off day.

Health Risks Associated with Surgery

Prostate cancer surgery may lead to erectile dysfunction, incontinence,[4] inguinal hernia, [5,6] penis shortening [7,8,9] and a host of other problems. Surgery of any kind including open and robotic surgery for prostate cancer carries with it serious health risks such as:

1. Impotence
2. Incontinence (urinary and fecal)
3. Heart Attack
4. Stroke
5. Blood Clots
6. Infection
7. Shortened length of penis
8. Death (rare)

Summary on Surgery

Surgery, including robotic surgery, is the most commonly provided treatment for prostate cancer even though according to most available literature not associated with these procedures, it has the greatest risks of the most serious side effects of all prostate cancer treatments.

Conventional Photon Radiation

Radiation therapy is an option for men with any stage of prostate cancer. There are two main types of radiation therapy - conventional photon radiation, discussed in the first part of this section, and proton therapy discussed in the latter part of this section. Men with early stage prostate cancer may choose radiation therapy instead of surgery. Radiation may also be used after surgery to destroy any cancer cells that remain in the previously treated area. Radiation treatment may be used to help relieve pain in later stages of prostate cancer.

The most common type of radiation is conventional photon radiation therapy. This type of radiation has been around for a long time and uses high-energy rays similar to what is used in Xray machines to kill prostate cancer cells. Doctors use several types of conventional photon radiation therapy to treat prostate cancer and some men receive one or more of the different types of radiation. In treatment of prostate cancer this type of radiation is normally administered externally with the most common approach now being the use of Intensity Modulated Radiation Therapy (IMRT) which will be discussed shortly. Another way of administering this radiation is internally in which radioactive "seeds" are implanted in the prostate to kill cancer cells located there. Proton therapy is newer type of external radiation that is significantly different from the conventional photon radiation and is gaining in popularity.

Intensity Modulated Radiation Therapy

External-beam radiation therapy is most often delivered in the form of conventional photon beams, the basic unit of light and other forms of electromagnetic radiation and can be thought of as a bundle of energy. The amount of energy in a photon can vary. For example, the photons in gamma rays have the highest energy, followed by the photons in x-rays.

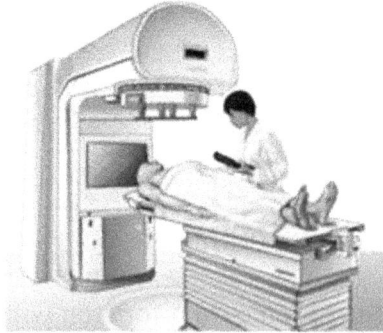

Many types of external-beam radiation therapy are delivered using a machine called a linear accelerator (also called a LINAC). A LINAC uses electricity to form a stream of fast moving subatomic particles. This creates high-energy radiation that may be used to treat cancer. National Cancer Institute

In conventional photon radiation treatment, radiation is directed to the prostate cancer from an outside source. An unfortunate aspect of conventional photon radiation is that as the radiation enters the body its strongest dose hits the tissue in front of the prostate. Since the level of radiation has to be strong enough to kill cancer, the dosage is usually higher where it enters the body so that as it loses power, it still has enough energy to kill the cancer in the prostate. Furthermore, conventional photon radiation does not stop when it hits the prostate but continues on through the body possibly harming normal healthy tissue in the process. In conventional photon radiation a broad beam of radiation is directed to the cancer site and normal healthy tissue is not excluded.

With many of the concerns conventional photon radiation has, a new and increasingly popular variant of conventional external photon radiation is Intensity Modulated Radiation Therapy (IMRT), which reduces some of the side effects with this type of radiation. This approach is an effort to control the dosage of radiation normal healthy tissue receives. This is achieved by the multidimensional delivery of the conventional photon radiation using hundreds of tiny radiation beam-shaping devices, called collimators, to deliver a single dose of radiation so that each directional beam of radiation hits the site of the cancer, thereby increasing its ability to kill cancer cells. Delivering this type of radiation to the prostate comes in from a number of different angles in an effort to minimize radiation exposure to normal healthy tissue. This approach is a significant improvement in the delivery of conventional photon radiation and is now the second most common approach to treating prostate cancer. Keeping the dose of radiation to healthy tissue low and high at the tumor can deliver IMRT with fewer side effects than non-IMRT conventional photon radiation. The side effects of IMRT are still the same as those of conventional photon radiation therapy but occur less frequently and with less intensity. Recent advancements in IMRT have further reduced the risks of some of the erectile problems that result from radiation.

Side Effects Risks

Many of the concerns of the earlier conventional photon radiation such as the high amount of radiation still exist for its newer method of delivery such as IMRT.

1. While the newer variant of IMRT has fewer side effects than the earlier methods of delivery, one critical issue is that it can take longer to deliver IMRT, up to 20 minutes.
2. This longer period of delivery deposits more radiation into the body that is spread around a large amount of normal tissue increasing the risk of secondary cancer. While side effects are less with the latest variants of IMRT, some men may also experience lasting bowel and urinary problems.
3. Conventional photon radiation in IMRT and other applications also have a significantly higher chance of causing secondary cancer caused by the radiation itself.

Internal Conventional Photon Radiation– Brachytherapy

In this approach small seeds are implanted in the prostate that release radiation on an ongoing basis. This radiation kills cancer cells while not harming normal cells. Since there have been reports of one or more seeds traveling to different parts of the body the current approach is to implant the seeds attached to one another on a strand or string. Dozens of seeds are injected into the prostate and surrounding area. The seeds are first of all placed inside needles that are then inserted into the prostate. When the needles are removed, the string or strand of seeds remains behind. The injected seeds release radiation for months and do not need to be removed once the radiation is gone. The process is usually done in one day and the patient then resumes his normal life.

Side Effect Risks

1. Urinary problems such as incontinence.
2. Rectal scarring
3. Sexual problems such as impotence

Proton Radiation Therapy

The most promising type of external radiation is proton therapy. This treatment differs significantly from conventional external radiation treatment in that it involves delivery of a stronger dose of radiation directly to the cancer with minimal harm to healthy tissue. Protons are a type of charged particle. Using medical physics the proton beam is accelerated to close to 300,000 miles per second and is manipulated so that it passes into your body with minimal harm being done to normal tissue until it reaches the cancer where it then unleashes its full power and then totally dissipates. Unlike conventional photon radiation, proton therapy does not continue on past the targeted cancer thus sparing healthy tissue from exit damage.

Due to their relatively large mass, protons have little lateral side scatter in the tissue; the beam does not broaden much, stays focused on the tumor shape, and delivers only low-dose side-effects to surrounding tissue. All protons of a given energy have a certain range and very few protons penetrate beyond that distance. The result is that the bulk of the dose of radiation is primarily delivered to the targeted cancer tumor with minimal damage to non-cancerous tissue. The important fact to understand about proton therapy is that it uses one-third of the amount of radiation used in conventional photon radiation and most of that radiation is deposited directly into the cancerous tumor.

A Layman's Explanation of the differences between Conventional Photon Radiation Versus Proton Radiation

It is very important to understand the difference between conventional photon radiation and proton therapy. Fully understanding this crucial difference allows a man to make a more informed decision about which treatment to select to destroy his prostate cancer. Not possessing such an understanding is dangerous in that it makes us vulnerable to follow treatment recommendations that will generate adverse side effects that could have been avoided.

The big difference between conventional photon radiation and proton therapy radiation lies in the way they deposit energy in living tissue. With photons energy is deposited in small packets all along its path as it passes through tissue. In proton therapy most of their energy is deposited at the end of their path where the cancer is located and very little is deposited along the way. This process is referred to as the Bragg peak and is the key feature of proton radiation and is shown in the graph below.

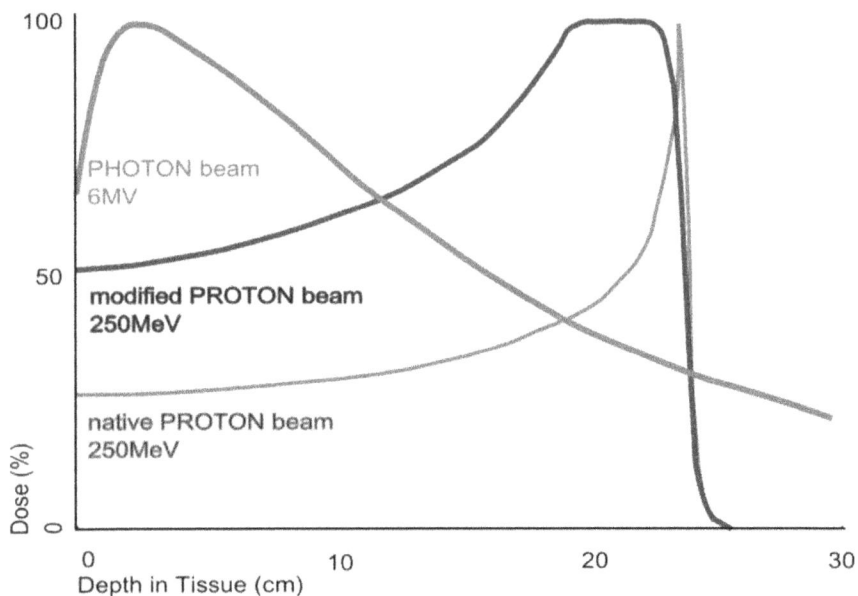

This graph shows the ability of the proton beam to pass into tissue and go to a depth where the tumor is before releasing its bundle of energy. The above graph shows the photon beam releasing its bundle of energy as soon as it enters the body and gradually weakening until it reaches the tumor at 20 cm of depth into your body and continues releasing energy until it passes through the rest of your body. The modified proton beam is shown with it being manipulated to release little or no energy until it reaches the tumor at 20 cm where it discharges all of its energy and goes no further. This modified proton beam in used in treatment. The native proton beam is not used in treatment and simply shows the path of an unmodified proton beam.

The Manipulation of Conventional Photon Radiation versus Proton Therapy Radiation

When radiation is used to treat cancer it can be thought of as a bundle of energy that is delivered to the human body. In treating prostate cancer this bundle of energy from either conventional photon radiation or proton therapy radiation is delivered over a five to nine week period of time. The goal of this delivery of energy is selective cell destruction intended to destroy cancer cells, a process called apoptosis, while minimizing harm to non-cancerous cells. It is the significant difference in how this bundle of energy is delivered via conventional photon radiation versus proton therapy radiation that account for its ability to destroy cancer cells while not harming healthy, non-cancerous cells. A good way of looking at the difference between conventional photon radiation versus proton radiation therapy is to focus on the three variables of (1) degree of spread, (2) ability to penetrate to specific depths, and (3) ability to completely discharge its energy at a specified location.

Controlling Where the Bundle of Radiation Energy Goes

While conventional photon radiation cannot be easily manipulated, proton therapy radiation can be controlled in several ways. One is by directing where it goes. This bundle of energy remains focused and can then be directed to a specific location in the body with minimal scatter radiation going elsewhere. As this beam of energy leaves the linear accelerator it travels to the proton therapy machine where it passes through a brass device with an opening patterned after the shape of our prostate. One of these brass plates is made for the left side of our body and another one is made for the right side of our body. Each brass plate shapes the bundle of energy to enter the body at a point where it will travel to the prostate. There is minimal scatter or spillover radiation; so healthy, non-cancerous cells are not harmed.

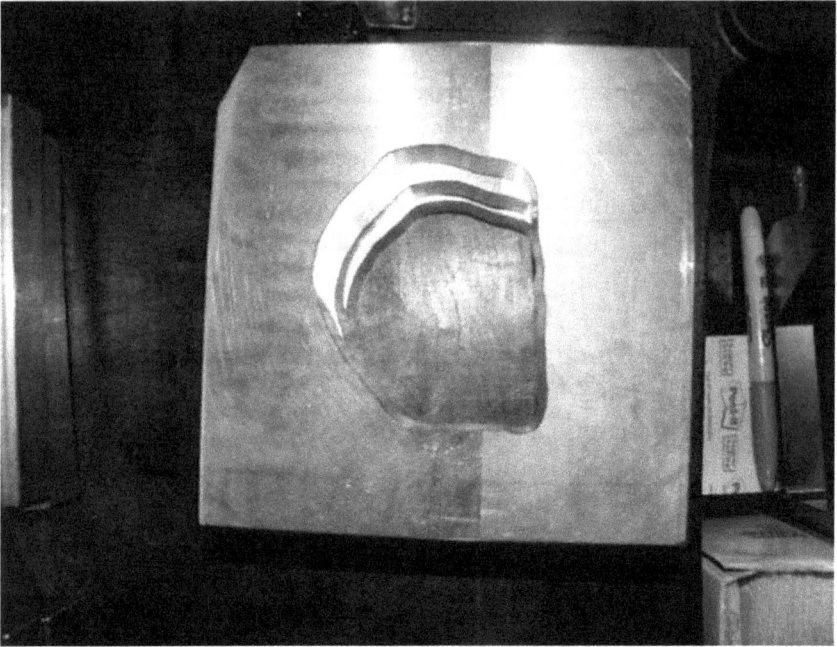

Right and left side brass-like plates shaped for my prostate

An analogy of how conventional photon radiation versus proton radiation works would be an example of a sheep herder observing a wolf killing one of his/her sheep. Assume that the sheepherder has the choice of using a shotgun or a rifle to kill the wolf. If he fired the shotgun at the wolf the chances are that he would kill the wolf. But in killing the wolf using the shotgun the sheepherder will likely also kill some of his sheep as well because of the scatter of the shotgun pellets causing collateral damage. If, instead, the sheepherder, elected to use the rifle he would likely be able to kill the wolf without killing any of his sheep. He would be able to do this by the greater control he would have in delivering the bullet directly to his intended target while doing minimal collateral damage. Proton beam radiation is like using the high-powered rifle to kill the wolf while conventional photon beam radiation is like using a shotgun to kill the wolf.

How proton radiation differs from conventional photon radiation is also evident in the difference between a floodlight and a hand held spotlight.

Controlling the Depth Where the Energy is Deposited

The proton therapy radiation beam is accelerated to such high speeds that it stays intact as it passes through our body until it reaches the tumor where it is programmed to stop and discharge all of its energy. Unlike conventional photon radiation, proton therapy radiation does not continue on through our body releasing additional energy until it finally passes through. Medical physicists and physicians calculate the density of tissue the beam of energy travels through and accelerate the bundle of radiation energy so that as it passes through human tissue it will only discharge its energy when it reaches the tumor. Proton therapy radiation is able to keep its energy until it reaches the tumor where it is then fully discharged. In addition to allowing for deeper penetration into tissue, linear accelerators provide a beam of proton therapy radiation energy with more sharply delineated borders. This, in turn, allows for higher doses of radiation to be directed at the prostate, seminal vesicles, and regional lymph nodes without harming healthy, non-cancerous tissue.

Side Effects of Proton Therapy Radiation

1. Low risk of fatigue during treatment.
2. Low possibility of burning while urination during middle part of treatment.
3. Low risk of erectile problems among men who had good erectile ability prior to treatment.
4. Low risks of a brief period of minor rectal bleeding shortly after treatment.
5. Very Low risk of secondary cancer.
6. Very low risk of rectal and urinary incontinence.

According to a report in Science Daily, proton beam therapy has minimal side effects and can be safely delivered to men with prostate cancer.[10] This article reported a study presented November 2, 2009, at the American Society for Radiation Oncology's 51st Annual Meeting in Chicago that found minimal urinary and rectal problems were evident in men having completed proton beam radiation for prostate cancer. With continuing research it is becoming increasing clear that proton therapy radiation treatment of prostate cancer has few serious side effects.

In my experience in going through the treatment with 100 or so other men, I heard few reports of any negative side effects attributable to proton therapy. One male friend reported a burning sensation when urinating for a temporary period of time and a few other men reported temporary fatigue. I personally have never experienced any negative side effect from proton therapy. The medical staff at the proton therapy center did alert us that we might experience rectal scarring around three months after treatment. This scarring may lead to a brief period of mild rectal bleeding. At the time this book was published it was slightly over a year since I completed treatment and I have never experienced any rectal problems. Only one of the men who went through treatment with me reported a brief period of minor rectal bleeding that lasted only a few days. I have never heard any reports of any other patient experiencing this side effect although I suspect some have experienced it. Side effects related directly to proton therapy are few. It can safely be said that any side effects are minimal in nature and brief in duration.

Significantly Less Secondary Cancer with Proton Radiation Compared to Conventional Photon Radiation

Another importance difference between conventional photon radiation and proton therapy radiation is in the different amount of radiation each discharges into our body. Radiation in any form is capable of causing cancer if enough of it is experienced. Conventional photon radiation uses around 66% more radiation to treat prostate cancer than proton therapy radiation. Prostate cancer patients treated with conventional photon radiation thus have a significantly higher incidence of radiation side effects such as burns to the rectum and urethra along with a significantly higher risk of causing secondary cancer. Research was presented in September of 2008 at the 50th Annual Meeting of the American Society for Therapeutic Radiology and Oncology in Boston reported that over a 26 year time period the risk for developing secondary cancer is 50% less when proton therapy radiation is used compared to when conventional photon radiation is used.[11] The greater degree of radiation and the diffuse way patients are exposed to it in conventional photon radiation therapy poses a significantly higher risk for developing secondary cancer than proton therapy radiation. The greater precision of proton therapy allows significantly less radiation to go to the bladder and rectum thereby reducing urinary and rectal side effects. Proton therapy may decrease the rates of secondary cancer caused by radiation by up to 30-40% compared to IMRT.

Some disadvantages of IMRT include keeping the beam on the target with more spillover radiation spreading to surrounding healthy tissue. There is also more radiation delivered overall which may result in a higher body dose. Unlike proton radiation, which is delivered in around 10 seconds, IMRT radiation can take around 20 minutes leading to over 60% greater exposure to radiation.

Treatment Comparisons of Surgery, Conventional Photon Radiation and Proton Therapy

Treatment Comparison	Proton Therapy	Conventional Photon Radiation	Surgery
Non-Invasive	*Yes*	*Yes*	*No*
Outpatient	*Yes*	*Yes*	*No*
Risk of Impotency	*Low*	*Moderate*	*Moderate to High*
Risk of Incontinence	*Low*	*Moderate*	*Moderate*
Risk of Healthy Tissue Damage	*Low*	*Moderate*	*Moderate*
Risk of Secondary Cancer	*Extremely Low*	*Low*	*Low*
Risk of Having to Repeat Treatment	*Low*	*Low to Moderate*	*Low*

Other Treatments

The focus in this Chapter has been comparing and contrasting the three most widely used treatments of prostate cancer, surgery, conventional photon radiation delivered via brachytherapy or IMRT, and proton therapy radiation. Since hormone therapy and chemotherapy are sometimes used in conjunction with the other treatments they will only be briefly discussed. Those of you seeking more information on the different treatments for prostate cancer are encouraged to visit the website of the American Cancer Society and the National Cancer Institute.

Hormone Therapy Surgery

Orchiectomy: Since male hormones (androgens) can cause prostate cancer to grow, efforts have long been directed at stopping them. Since the testicles are the body's main source of the male hormone androgen, one procedure that has never gained popularity but is still used in some instances is the surgical removal of the testicles identified as orchiectomy. This procedure is rarely used today and has been largely replaced by drugs to suppress the male hormones.

Hormone Suppressant Therapy

One of the causes of prostate cancer is the presence of male hormones. The rationale behind hormone suppressant therapy is to use female hormones to reduce or eliminate the presence of male hormones and thus stop feeding the cancer. Hormone therapy can be used by itself or in combination with other treatments. It is also commonly used to treat prostate cancer that reappears after treatment. This approach works by the hormone keeping prostate cancer cells from receiving the male hormones necessary for them to grow.

Drugs commonly used in hormone therapy are luteining hormone-releasing hormone agonists: These are drugs that stop the testicles from producing testosterone. Trade names of such drugs include leuprolide, tritorlin, and goserelin. These drugs are also referred to as gonadotropin-releasing hormone agonists.

Antiandrogens: Additional drugs that are also sometimes used to block the action of male hormones and include trade names such as flutamide, nilutamide, and bicalutamide.

Other drugs used in hormone therapy to stop action of male hormones include ketoconazole and aminoglutethimide.

If you have spent any time at all around middle aged women going through menopause, you will be familiar with some of the side effect of hormone therapy such as hot flashes and loss of sexual desire. Another negative side effect of lowering your male hormones is that it may lead to impotence and a loss of libido as well as also weakening your bones making you more prone to fractures. If you have osteopenia or osteoporosis you need to discuss this negative side effect with your physician before starting on hormone therapy. Sometimes men on hormone therapy experience what is referred to as a "flare up" where the side effects become especially pronounced. In addition, weight gain may accompany hormone therapy especially evident in belly fat around your waist. Other issues your physician needs to monitor are increased risk of diabetes and possible increase in your cholesterol levels. When cancer has spread to other parts of the body, hormone therapy becomes the main treatments.

Side Effects

1. Hot flashes.
2. Loss of sexual desire.
3. Breasts enlargement.
4. Weight gain
5. Increased risk of breast cancer

Chemotherapy

When cancer has spread to other parts of the body and hormone therapy is no longer controlling it, chemotherapy is employed. Chemotherapy involves the use of powerful drugs to kill cancer cells. These drugs are usually administered intravenously by injection either at a clinic or your physician's office. They are frequently given in conjunction with one or more other treatments.

Side Effects

1. Lowering of your red blood cells
2. Loss of hair (it usually grows back).
3. Digestive problems such as vomiting, diarrhea, and nausea
4. Poor appetite.

Cryrotherapy

In this procedure, the cancer tumor is frozen which kills the cancer cells. A device is inserted through the scrotum to where the prostate is located and drops the temperature to freezing in that area. Warm saline water is circulated through a catheter to protect nearby healthy tissue. Unfortunately, normal non-cancerous cells may also be destroyed in the process. Some experts recommend cryrotherapy for second treatment interventions after prostate cancer has returned.

Side Effects

Side effects are similar to those experienced from surgery and conventional photon radiation.
1. Sexual problems
2. Incontinence
3. Other problems.

High Intensity Focused Ultrasound (HIFU)

Using high intensity focused ultrasound is possible to increase the temperature inside the prostate by as much as 85° Celsius using a focused ultrasound beam which can kill cancer cells while not harming healthy tissue. This procedure works by inserting a probe into the rectum after a spinal or epidural anesthesia has been given. A beam of high intensity focused ultrasound is then emitted from this probe. The sudden and intense absorption of the ultrasound beam rapidly increases the temperature destroying the cancer cells. The area destroyed by each beam is very small and specific. The treatment can take between two to three hours. One treatment is usually sufficient to destroy the prostate cancer. By repeating the process and moving the focal point it is possible to destroy the prostate tissue. The treatment is usually performed on an outpatient basis.

High-intensity focused ultrasound (HIFU) is emerging as a promising treatment for localized prostate cancer treatment. HIFU therapy is noninvasive with minimal side effects. There have been ongoing concerns HIFU may induce mechanical damage that could lead to the dissemination of cancer cells into the blood leading to distant metastasis. Recent research suggests that this risk is minimal.

HIFU is not approved in the United States so men seeking this treatment for their prostate cancer they have to go to other countries where it is permitted.

Side Effects

1. Erectile problems.
2. Bowel problems
3. Low risk of incontinence

Conclusion

Making an informed and educated choice of treatment for your prostate cancer is of crucial importance. Like it or not, after you have been diagnosed with prostate cancer, you may not only be in a battle for your life, if you go through treatment you will be battling for a life with the highest quality possible. Next to heart disease and lung cancer, untreated prostate cancer is the biggest killer of men. Like anyone involved in mortal combat, be it in a warlike setting facing enemy combatants or battling prostate cancer, we not only have to select the best weapons we can find but to also keep our spirits high.

Living without enjoyable sex or being unable to control your urine clearly lowers the quality of our life. Fecal incontinence can be even more distressing. I have actually encountered men who were so embittered from what they described as the horrible side effects from surgery and conventional photon radiation, they stated they would have forgone treatment altogether and taken their chances with untreated prostate cancer.

This review of prostate cancer treatments is preliminary in nature. You are encouraged to seek more detailed information from the American Cancer Society and the National Cancer Institute's websites. At this point it is your responsibility to educate yourself sufficiently so that you can make an informed decision in selecting the treatment that best meets your needs.

Chapter Five

Selecting Proton Therapy

"Upside: No pain at all and effective. Fewest side effects the worst of which is possible fatigue. Unlike very common x-ray radiation it only affects the cancerous area not all the nearby body tissues."

Comments of a Proton Therapy patient
from Protonpals.net website

Proton Therapy - Leading the Charge in the War on Cancer

The world's largest medical complex, the Texas Medical Center, is located in the bustling city of Houston, Texas. Literally a city within a city, close to 100,000 people work there providing over six million patient care visits annually. With more than 49 medical related facilities covering over 1000 acres, the Texas Medical Center is the greatest concentration of health care providers that have ever been amassed in one location. Thirteen hospitals, two medical schools, four nursing schools, plus schools of dentistry, pharmacy, public health and other advanced degree granting institutions make up the Texas Medical Center. Larger than the size of downtown Dallas, it draws over 160,000 daily visitors and over six million annual patient visitors. With over 20,000 physicians and advanced degreed health care professionals, The Texas Medical Center provides some of the best care available anywhere. And within this center lies the world's leading cancer treatment center, the University of Texas's M.D. Anderson Cancer Center.

The M.D. Anderson Cancer Center has been ranked for years as the number one cancer treatment center in America by U.S. News and

World Report.[1] Employing close to 18,000 people and providing care to over 100,000 patients annually, M.D. Anderson is in the forefront in this war on cancer. The good news in this war is that the tide is turning for the better as more and more people are surviving cancer and going on to live full, productive lives. Among these survivors is a small but rapidly growing group of cancer fighters who are achieving some of the greatest successes in this war. The battle site is the MD Anderson Proton Therapy Center and it is here where one of the single greatest weapons against encapsulated cancer is being used with tremendous success, proton therapy.

Providing prostate cancer treatment since 2006, the Proton Therapy Center has a steadily growing list of graduates from its treatment who are relatively free of adverse side effects and, most importantly, experiencing a degree of treatment success in terms of remaining free from cancer that is as good if not better than any other treatment. Soon, the Proton Therapy Center will release its own follow-up data and the medical community and world in general will be better able to judge its effectiveness. There are a growing number of proton therapy center across America. Please check in Appendix C for a listing of the over 12 proton therapy centers that are now operating or under development in America plus one in Korea and another in Germany.

There's something else that's happening in the proton therapy treatment program that is not related to its nuclear accelerator or other medical aspects of the treatment. It is something so subtle it is overlooked yet its importance in treatment cannot be dismissed. What is going on is a powerful social bonding process among the patients as they go through the 39 treatment sessions together. The way the treatment program is set up each day, usually at the same time and location, a small group of patients undress and put on their surgical gowns, prepare for treatment, and sit in a changing/waiting area socializing with one another. As this daily routine goes on for eight weeks of treatment they get to know one another and a strong social bond of friendship develops. Every aspect of their prostate cancer and its treatment is repeatedly discussed amid joking and kidding and, as this goes on, much of their fear and trepidation associated with their cancer melts away. Included in this mixture is an active fraternal organization of former patients, ProtonPals. With weekly group dinners together at local restaurants, another powerful effective adjunct is added to their prostate cancer treatment. The resultant patient support generates one of the most powerful types of the widely recognized health enhancer - social support. The bonding together of a small group of men into a tight supportive group is as crucial in the field of health care as it is in the military.

What follows next is my story of going through prostate cancer at the proton therapy center and not only eliminating my cancer with no side effects but also developing some of the best friendships I've ever developed in such a short period of time. This adjunctive social aspect of going through daily treatment with a large number of other men was an unexpected bonus. My conclusion from this experience is not only that proton therapy works but that the even greater facilitation of the support that naturally forms among men going through protracted treatment together can add to its effectiveness by improving the level of life satisfaction experienced during treatment.

In any battle, weapons are a crucial part of winning the war. Generally speaking, the better the weapons are, the greater the likelihood of success in a war. But a high level of support and camaraderie among members of the fighting group, the Esprit de Corps, also contributes to success in combat. Proton therapy is the single best weapon in the battle of prostate cancer and its effectiveness is increased with this added social support.

I first became aware of the remarkable degree of camaraderie among men going through proton therapy for prostate cancer from reading online reports from legitimate grass root patient organizations such as the fraternal groups of former proton therapy patients the Brotherhood of the Balloon (ProtonBob.com) and Protonpals.net. From visiting their websites and reading their extensive blogs, it was evident that strong friendships developed during treatment along with a desire among some of the men to keep those rewarding associations alive by joining one of the proton therapy support groups. I saw the likelihood of my participating in such a fraternal bond as another reason for going to the proton therapy center at MD Anderson. Once I selected proton beam treatment I contacted the MD Anderson Cancer Center in Houston, Texas for information about their proton beam treatment program for prostate cancer. What began next was the start of my incredible journey.

My Choice - The MD Anderson Proton Center

"Hello, this is Yvette Ranson (a pseudonym), may I help you," the friendly voice with an interesting accent stated on the other end of the phone.

Identifying myself, I replied that I had recently been diagnosed with prostate cancer and was seeking information about their proton treatment for it.

"We will be glad to send you information and to also provide a second opinion if that is what you are seeking," Yvette replied as I found myself trying to figure out her accent.

"Yes, I would like to get a second opinion and to see if your proton therapy is appropriate for me," I replied as I thought to myself that she was German based on her accent. I thanked her and hung up.

I completed the forms Yvette sent and signed releases of my medical information so all of my medical records could be sent to MD Anderson. I also had the original biopsy slides sent as well as they had requested.

A week later the friendly voice of Yvette called back. "Mr. Dawley, we have you scheduled to see Dr. Brown at 12:00 PM on 1-6-11."

Pleased at getting an early appointment, I thanked Yvette and told her I liked her accent asking, "Are you of German ancestry?"

Yvette laughed and replied she was from Jamaica.

My exchange with Yvette was pleasant. She related in a warm, sincere, and caring manner. I soon discovered this attitude was characteristic of the vast majority of employees at MD Anderson.

Arriving the day before my appointment, my wife and I checked into a nearby motel and went for my appointment at the Proton Center the following morning. The building housing the Proton Center is an impressive futuristic-looking structure with a two-story large glass-paneled facade on the front right side.

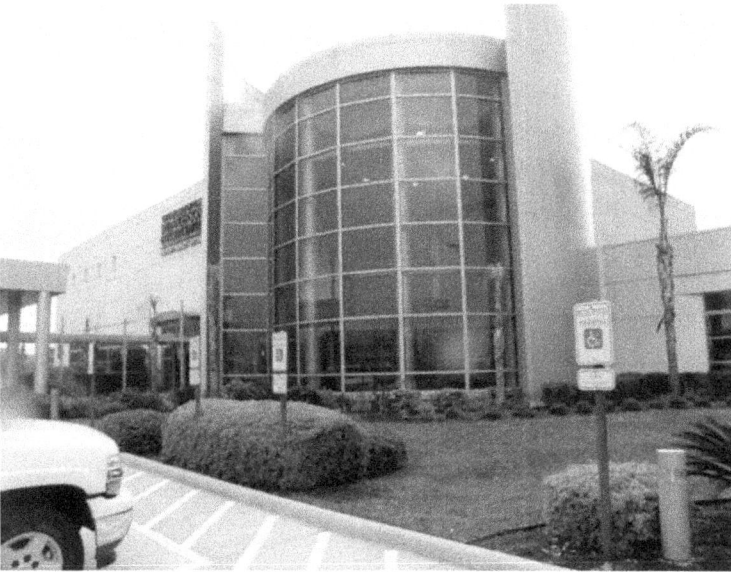

Proton Therapy Center at M.D. Anderson Cancer Center, Houston, Texas

Walking into the Proton Center I noticed how the large glass circular façade stood out catching one's attention. As we walked into the Proton Center I looked at the wide winding stairway going downstairs beside that large glass façade.

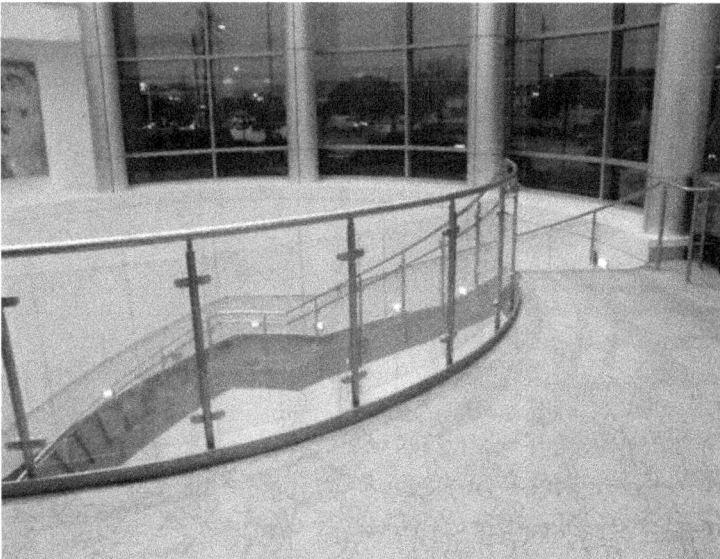

PHOTO of Stairway

What's down there, I wondered, a curiosity that was to increase in the coming weeks.

As we walked in a man around my age was joking with the young woman receptionist. Another man of similar age was talking in a friendly manner with the hospital police officer stationed at the center. Groups of other men and a few women and children were also in the waiting room or coming or going downstairs. All seemed relaxed and at ease with one another.

"Mr. Harold Dawley, "the voiced called out after being seated in the reception area for ten minutes.

Another friendly female employee led me into a small treatment room. I first filled out paper work, gave a blood sample, had my vitals taken and was then placed in a small treatment room and told that my treatment team would soon meet with me.

Shortly thereafter, a knock on the door was followed by the entry of a smiling young woman.

"I'm Carla (a pseudonym), Dr. Brown's (a pseudonym) nurse and I will be your nurse if you go through treatment here.

More paperwork and Carla provided information on the proton beam treatment of prostate cancer.

After 20 minutes, another knock and another smiling female face came to the door.

"Hello, I'm Doris (a pseudonym), and I am the Nurse Practitioner that works with Dr. Brown. I will work with you if you receive treatment here."

Doris provided more information about what to expect going through treatment. She then added that engaging in sex at least three to five times a week during treatment would help maintain the blood vessels feeding nerves in my penis associated with experiencing satisfaction in sex remain in good shape. She added that doing so would reduce the chances of my experiencing erectile problems later on.

"There are obviously no guarantees to you or any man your age that you won't experience erectile dysfunction as you age. We've found that men who engage in sex three to five times a week seem to do better," Doris added.

Next, a small slender woman who looked like she just graduated from high school walked in and introduced herself as Dr. Brown (a pseudonym).

"Hello Mr. and Mrs. Dawley. If you elect to receive proton therapy treatment here I will be your doctor."

Dr. Brown spent twenty minutes or so providing further information about proton therapy treatment for prostate cancer. She added that some men's prostates are too large and that they would have to go on hormone therapy for a while in order to shrink it. She indicated that my prostate size was OK. She then asked me about my sexual functioning, which was good, with no erectile or ejaculatory problems.

"Good," Dr. Brown stated.

"Your PSA is low, your Gleason score is a 6, and your staging is a T2B all of which point to a good prognosis for your treatment success. You are a good candidate for proton therapy," Dr. Brown added.

"We do need to do a repeat MRI because the one your doctor did showed some suspicious area near your lymph nodes. I can have it scheduled right away so we can get the results tomorrow."

Linda and I exchanged concerned looks as the words suspicious area resonated in our heads.

Sure enough, in less than ten minutes Dr. Brown had scheduled an MRI for me the following morning.

"Go ahead and have the EndoRectal MRI done and I will see you tomorrow afternoon," Dr. Brown stated.

I didn't like the sound of the term "Endo-rectal" and images of a large object going into my rectum came to my mind along with a feeling of apprehension.

I took an enema the morning of the MRI and reported for this test. By the time I got there my apprehension about an "endorectal MRI" had grown to a state of mild anxiety.

I was led to a small changing room and told to take everything off the lower part of my body and put on a surgical gown with the back open.

I know why they want the back open, I thought to myself with a growing sense of unease.

Finally a young woman appeared and asked "Are you Harold Dawley?" as she looked on my photo wristband that had earlier been placed on me.

"Do you know why you are here and what we are going to do?", she asked.

In a feeble attempt at humor to reduce my rising anxiety, I replied, "You're going to stick something up my rectum?"

The young woman laughed comfortably and then reassured me by adding "Trust, me it won't be unpleasant."

The young woman then led me into the MRI room where another young woman was standing with two other women who looked like students.

With my eyes furtively scanning the room for any dangerous looking projectile that could be inserted into my rectum, the technician told me to try to relax. She then stated, "Mr. Dawley, I am first going to insert some pain deadeners and lubricant into your rectum and will then ask you to lie down on a treatment gantry in front of the MRI machine with your back side exposed."

Why do I need pain deadeners, I worried.

Doing as she had requested, the first woman then deftly inserted some type of liquid into my rectum before I realized what was going on.

"Just lie there and relax for a minute or two Mr. Dawley while we prepare for the examination."

The first woman then discussed with the other three women what they would be doing.

Definitely students, I thought to myself as I self-consciously lay there with my naked backside exposed to them.

Trying to control my anxiety, I was thinking positive thoughts and breathing deeply when the first woman asked;

"Do you have any questions before we begin," she asked.

Pausing, I didn't know what to say. I am not good at telling jokes but since my first feeble attempt at humor had made her laugh before and helped to relax me, I gave it another try.

"What happens if I have thoughts of a sexual nature when you do whatever you are going to do."

Laughter burst out among the four women as they all enjoyed my little bit of humor. I relaxed a bit and before I knew what was happening, the first woman quickly and skillfully inserted an object into my rectum.

"You are doing fine, Mr. Dawley, just breathe deeply and relax," she reassured me.

Within a short period of time the MRI was finished and, to my relief, the object was removed from my rectum. She was right; it wasn't that bad.

Linda and I went out to eat that night at a nice restaurant and we both slept soundly.

When we met with Dr. Brown the following morning she got right down to business.

"The MRI indicates that your cancer is still encapsulated within your prostate and that is good. But the report indicates that your lymph nodes are enlarged and it recommends a MRI guided needle biopsy be done to see what is in them."

Alarm bells started going off in our heads as Linda and I looked at each other.

"What could be in there?" I asked knowing full well the suspicion was that it might be cancer.

Dr. Brown replied "We really don't know. With your level of cancer I don't think we need to worry about it. Let's just go ahead and get it done and find out."

Not satisfied or reassured I continued, "What if they find cancer there – will I still be a candidate for proton therapy?"

"Not initially. If there is cancer in them, and I really doubt that there is, we will simply use a different treatment plan to treat your prostate cancer."

I was somewhat reassured but I could tell Linda was still very alarmed.

"Will his cancer be curable if it has spread to his lymph nodes" Linda besieged Dr. Brown.

"All we can do is find out what the pathology report has to say," Dr. Brown stated.

About a week later Linda and I were back at MD Anderson for the needle biopsy.

It's funny how little things can stick in your mind. What had stuck in my mind was the image of someone leaning over me and sticking a big needle in my belly probing for my enlarged lymph nodes.

Arriving for the procedure, I was led to a changing room, told to undress from the waist down, and to put on a surgical gown.

A friendly male nurse who took my vitals interviewed me. I jokingly asked him how big was the needle they were going to stick into my belly.

He laughed and said it won't be bad, adding "Plus you will have waking sedation."

Since that sounded like I wouldn't feel the needle going deep into my stomach, I relaxed a bit.

Next, a young man arrived dressed in surgical scrubs and identified himself as a resident working with the physician who was going to do the needle biopsy. He carefully explained the procedure I was about to receive. I felt further relieved by what he said.

Then, a drip was inserted into one of my veins and a sedative administered. After a few minutes, I was wheeled into the MRI room.

A young oriental woman came up and introduced herself as the doctor who was going to be doing the needle biopsy. She told me my lymph nodes had shrunk and it may not be possible to get a tissue sample. Hearing that they had shrunk was reassuring.

Totally relaxed and at ease I watched as the physician leaned over my stomach and inserted the needle. I felt no pain or discomfort. After a moment or two she withdrew the needle and left.

Shortly she returned and told me she was able to get a good sample.

"Your doctor will go over the pathology results with you," the physician said as she left.

Two very anxiety laden weeks passed in which both Linda and I worried about the cancer having spread. I found myself going back to the initial process of accepting the possibility of death and that if my cancer was going to kill me I told myself I was lucky at having lived a good life. But these two weeks were clearly two of the toughest weeks Linda and I had to endure in my prostate cancer treatment.

Then the call came.

"Hello Mr. Dawley," the friendly voice of Dr. Brown was on the phone.

Intuitively I felt she had good news.

"The results of the MRI are negative. The cancer has not spread beyond your prostate. This means we can proceed with your treatment. Carla will soon send you an appointment time for your fiducial and simulation."

I asked her what was involved with these two procedures.

Dr. Brown replied that the fiducails involved the placement of two small brass markers on the prostate so that it could be easily identified to ensure the proton beam was delivered to where it needed to go. She added that simulation was the process of getting the proper alignment coordinates for my receiving the proton beam during treatment.

Two weeks later Linda and I were back in Houston. Checking into a motel, we called out for room service, bathed and went to bed early.

The next day my rectum got one hell of a workout.

First thing in the Wednesday morning of 2-16-11, I had to give myself an enema. I hate receiving an enema.

I then arrived at the clinic where the fiducails were to be done.

Soon I was placed in a small room with a smaller than usual treatment platform lined in padded vinyl. I was told to undress from the waist down and to put on one of the surgical gowns, open side to the back.

After I removed my trousers and underwear and put on the gown, the technician asked me to lay sideways on the table and sort of pull up my knees to my chest exposing my rectum for easy access.

I felt awkward, exposed, and vulnerable lying there in that position.

The technician told me to relax and that he was going to insert some lubricating fluid into my rectum adding that it also contained a pain deadener.

The question, *Why do I need a pain deadener* crossed my mind as alarm bells again started going off.

Before I knew it his rubber gloved finger was in my rectum and he was rubbing the liquid all around its inside.

Feeling stupid lying on that table with my knees pulled up and my rectum exposed, Dr. Brown walked in.

"How are you Mr. Dawley" she cheerfully asked.

"Fine" I replied wondering what was going to happen next.

"Mr. Dawley, I will soon enter your rectum with a small device that I will use to insert the fiducial markers on your prostate. You will feel a slight pitch but unlike a biopsy I will not be pulling out any tissue.

Breathing deeply and trying to relax my sphincter muscle as much as I could, I felt the device slowly slide into my rectum.

Some twisting and turning and moving the device around inside my rectum followed until Dr. Brown finally said "OK, Mr. Dawley you will soon feel a pinch.

I felt the pinch and it wasn't that bad.

More moving the device around in my rectum followed before Dr. Brown again stated she was going to insert another brass marker.

Then it was over and Dr. Brown slowly withdrew the device from my rectum.

That's enough rear end work to last me for a lifetime, I thought to myself hoping that nothing else was going to go in it.

"Good job, Mr. Dawley" Dr. Brown stated as she left.

As I walked out to the waiting room where Linda was waiting, I put on an air of bravado when she asked how it went.

"Nothing to it," I replied in a somewhat cavalier manner adding "It was a piece of cake."

We then went to back to the Proton Center where I was told to go downstairs.

I was flushed with excitement at the prospect of actually going downstairs!

Since my first arrival at the Proton Center I had been fascinated by what was at the bottom of those stairs. Fantastic images came to my mind such as big machines shooting a healing ray. I was excited as Linda and I headed for the descending stairs. Standing at the top of the stairs we looked down. We then descended and my prostate cancer treatment journey began.

As we walked downstairs I could see a large waiting room and several men my age. I also saw several children and an area where a number of children's toys were located. Several young women were also present. The presence of women and children surprised me because at that point I did not yet know that proton treatment is a major advancement in the treatment of a number of cancers including brain cancer, esophageal cancer, lung cancer, and even breast cancer. From there I saw several doors leading off to the right and to the left.

Looking at the large double glass doors I told myself, *that's where the proton beam is located.*

Shortly thereafter a medical technician came to the side door and called my name.

Leading me to a small changing room the technician stated "Please take off your clothes from the waist down and come out when you have put on one of the gowns placed on the bench, back open."

I had followed the advice given to me at various stages to try and drink a lot of water so my bladder was full. Having followed that advice conscientiously my bladder was so full I felt it could burst.

Dancing from one foot to the other, I told the technician that I had to let out some of my urine.

"Go ahead and let some out," he added.

The technician then led me to a large room that contained an MRI machine and some other machines.

"Please lay down Mr. Dawley."

As I lay down he placed a towel on my genital area and told me to raise my knees.

Oh boy, here we go again with more rear end work, I thought to myself as I cautiously raised my knees and tried to relax my sphincter muscle.

The technician then carefully explained that he was going to insert a small rubber balloon in my rectum. He added that this is what they will do for every treatment session.

Great, just what I don't want. I thought to myself.

"The idea of the balloon is to inflate it with water after it is inserted so that it will push your rectum away from your prostate that will receive the proton radiation. Also, by having a full bladder it will move your bladder away from your prostate and will hold your prostate in place so that we will be able to direct the radiation directly to it with minimal radiation hitting good, non-cancerous tissue," the technician stated.

Telling me to relax and to raise my legs, I felt the device delivering the balloon enter my rectum.

Boy do I hate having stuff shoved up my butt, I thought one more time as the technician skillfully inserted the device with minimal discomfort on my part.

"Now, Mr. Dawley I'm going to fill it with water and as I do you will feel a sense of fullness.

Sure enough, as he pumped in the water I felt my rectum expand. It was a sensation of getting ready to pass one huge stool.

After carefully lining me up on the machine and making a number of large x marks on my thighs, lower legs and stomach, he stated that proper alignment was crucial adding, "We will set your base alignment up now. Every time you receive proton treatment, your technician will make sure you are positioned identically to the way you are now positioned."

"I will take some X-ray images now and they will be used in the future to ensure the proton beam only goes to your prostate. These base measurements will be used in every treatment session to ensure you are properly aligned," the technician stated. He then stated that it was important for me to maintain my same weight as changing my weight during treatment by either gaining or losing five pounds or more would result in redoing the simulation.

I made a mental note to carefully monitor my weight.

The technician then passed a hand held sonogram over my bladder to see how much urine it held and then stated "You will need to let out more urine as your bladder is too full."

Taking a plastic cup, he drew a line near the top and then another line about a third of the way up from the top and stated "Fill this cup to this line with urine twice and then empty. Then fill it once to this bottom line and empty and come back."

When I got back on the MRI machine the technician again carefully lined me up.

"Dr. Brown will soon be here, Mr. Dawley."

"Hello Mr. Dawley," the cheerful voice of Dr. Brown filled the room. "You were real brave for the fiducails this morning."

"Thank you," I replied.

After checking my position the doctor and the technician left and entered the lead encased area as the MRI took several images.

After a minute or two, the technician entered the room and told me I had too much stool in my rectum and Dr. Brown wanted me to take an enema.

At this point all of the activity in my rectum and my intense dislike of giving myself an enema came to a head and I blurted out "I'm embarrassed to say it but at this point I don't think I can give myself an enema."

I immediately felt embarrassed and uncomfortable at having made the above statement.

"I fully understand Mr. Dawley; it is a common reaction among some of the men we see here.''

He then added in a kind voice "Would you like for me to give it to you?"

"Yes indeed I would, I just hate giving myself an enema."

After the enema I returned to the MRI room and the images were finished.

"You are all set to start your treatment Monday Mr. Dawley," Dr. Brown said as she walked out of the room. She then stated I should try to have a bowel movement every day before my treatment.

Before I left the MRI room the technician gave me a treatment schedule for the next eight weeks, a total of 39 sessions. A wave of relief and excitement swept over me as I was now ready to actually start my proton therapy.

Later that day my wife and I moved into the apartment we had leased for the duration of my treatment. It was a nice one-bedroom located in the Museum District of Houston.

It felt good to be in our new home away from home.

Chapter Six

Going Through Proton Therapy

"Approximately 33,000 patients have been treated worldwide with proton radiation, including cancer of the brain and spinal cord. The cure rate for prostate cancer is comparable to all other forms of treatment, and the side effect profile for erectile dysfunction and incontinence are lower. Many patients have had full post-treatment recovery, including myself."

Terry Wepsic, MD
Physician/Pathologist
Letter to the Editor
Wall Street Journal 2-1-05

Preparing for Proton Therapy

Linda and I settled into our comfortable furnished apartment at the Amalfi directly across the street from Herman Park and within walking distance of most of the Houston museums. We frequently would walk in the Park and there were several entertainment areas in the apartment complex where we had our friends over for wine and cheese parties. It was a lovely setting with landscaped yards and gardens. A large grocery store was three minutes away and a number of restaurants were also located nearby.

Lodging should not be a concern for anyone wishing to be treated at the Proton Therapy Center. Social work services are available to provide assistance in locating a suitable apartment with short-term leases. There are a large number of apartments available in the area around the Texas medical Center. Facilities are also available for those who want to bring their camper and stay in a campground. For those who have limited finances, M.D. Anderson also has small apartments available at reduced rates for its patients. Housing may also be available through local churches and charitable groups. If cost is not a major issue, I would suggest selecting an apartment in the Museum district near Herman Park. It is a lovely area with plenty of restaurants nearby. If you come in Mid February as we did you need to book an apartment in advance as the Rodeo is in town during that time and few apartments will be available near the Proton Therapy Center.

The Proton Therapy Center was a five-minute drive from our apartment. I quickly got used to the routine of awakening early for my treatment. Sometimes I would arrive early and stay late enjoying socializing with the other patients. Linda spent her days engaging in her hobby of going to thrift and consignment stores shopping for bargains. At least two or three times a week we would socialize with other patients by either going to dinner together, movies, or visiting our new friends at their apartments. I met the founder of Proton Pals, Joe Landry and got to know him and his lovely wife Marcia. One night Joe invited Linda and I to join him and Marcia to listen to Baroque classical music at an Episcopalian church in Herman Park.

It was a pleasant time.

I quickly got used to the routine of treatment. Each day began with my getting up around 4:30 AM for my 6:30 AM appointment. I would begin by drinking two or three cups of coffee as I found this increased the chances of having a bowel movement prior to treatment. It is important to have such a movement prior to treatment, because it may be difficult to insert the balloon and inflate it in your rectum if you don't. Plus, the stool may misalign your rectum from the original settings and require more adjustments prior to treatment.

The night before I started proton treatment I lay in bed with Linda talking about what to expect. I began by asking her if she thought I would hear a loud noise like a rifle shot. She responded by asking if I thought there would also be a flash of light like lightning striking. I responded by asking if I would feel it and if there would be any concussion from the proton beam.

Of course the above discussion was a humorous way of expressing our curiosity as to what it would be like experiencing proton treatment. Even though I had done a fair amount of research and felt I understood the basic concepts, I still thought about what it would be like actually going through treatment.

Would I feel the beam going in me, I wondered.

Going Through Proton Therapy

Monday morning, February 21, 2011 started off with a beautiful sunrise. Getting up at 4:30 AM, I was dressed and was ready to go by 5:30 AM. I drank my two cups of coffee and ate a small breakfast with Linda. Then, most importantly, I had a bowel movement. Finally at 5:45 we walked out to our car and drove to the Proton Therapy Center located less than five miles away. Pulling up, I stared again at the large glass facade and sensed excitement growing in me as I contemplated again going down the large winding stairway and actually starting my proton therapy.

What would treatment be like? I again wondered.

Entering the proton center, I signed in, something all patients do when they arrive. I then turned to Linda and I reached out and grabbed her hand and we began our descent to the floor below.

One of the most important journeys of my life was about to begin.

As we descended I quickly and excitedly looked around. Several men around my age sat at a small table and a number of young children and their parents were also present. We sat down near a small table and were joined by two men who had been sitting nearby. They smiled at us and said hello making us feel comfortable enough to begin talking with them. We discovered that one man was being treated for lung cancer while the other man was being treatment for esophageal cancer. They stated they had been referred to proton therapy as a last hope after all other treatments for their cancer had failed. Both looked in good health and indicated they were optimistic about beating their cancer.

Shortly thereafter, an attractive young woman came to the door "Mr. Harold Dawley?"

"Here" I responded and then accompanied her into the treatment areas.

"I'm Sara and I'm the technician who will be providing your treatment," she said in a pleasant voice as she smiled and held out her hand to me.

Leading me into the treatment area Sara went on to explain that each day when I arrived for my appointment I was to go directly to the patient changing area and take off the clothes on the lower half of my body and put on a gown. She added that it was important for me to stay hydrated by drinking water whenever I didn't feel I had a full bladder. She then added that if I felt the need for a bowel movement to go ahead and do so.

Upon reaching the patient changing area, there were two other men present. Both said hello to Sara and then introduced themselves to me. Sara showed me the locker and said, "I will be back to get you shortly."

The two men looked at me with curiosity and one asked with a slight smile on his face "Is this your first day?"

Smiling back I replied that it was my first day and then introduced myself and shook hands with them. Both were friendly and started giving me suggestions on what to do and what not to do as I went through proton therapy.

I then went about changing and the men resumed their discussion about fishing boats.

After I changed, I locked my clothes in a nearby locker and put the elastic band containing the key on my wrist. I then sat down and listened to the ongoing conversation.

One of the men told me to put on two gowns, one facing front and the other one facing back, "That way you will cover your backside and right before your treatment you can take off the second gown."

The other man asked me where I was from and how I found out about the Proton Center. I discovered that many of the men were curious how the other patients had found out about the proton center.

"I did research on the Internet and decided it was the treatment I wanted," I replied.

I had read reports on the Internet both at the Brotherhood of the balloon website (ProtonBob.com) and Protonpals.net about the remarkable camaraderie that formed among patients going through prostate cancer treatment at the proton center and was seeing it at the very beginning of my treatment.

"For most of us proton therapy was something our doctors did NOT recommend", one of the men added.

Several other men arrived and all began talking with one another in a friendly way. They were careful to involve me in their conversation and I felt welcomed and at ease.

"You will learn to feel when your bladder is at the right volume," one man stated and added, "It is better to be a little full instead of being too low."

Just then another man walked in, a black man who looked to be in his late 50's and the other men were pleased to see him. He turned out to be a natural born comedian and triggered belly laughter in all of us every day he came. He was our resident comedian until he graduated.

Spotting me again, Henry with a big smile on his face asked "Is this your first day?"

"Yes it is," I replied as I smiled back.

"Well, you may not know this but to celebrate it being your first day, they got a special balloon waiting for you."

Laughter broke out among the other men with Henry quickly joining in as he could no longer keep a straight face.

"I got that special balloon last week when they did my simulation," I replied and the laughter increased.

Any anxiety I had associated with treatment was immediately dissipated as the laughter soothed me.

Henry proved to be a one-man comedy show and kept all of us in stitches. We were lucky to go through treatment with him. I discovered that just about every time slot had one or more comedians present.

My First Treatment Session

In a short period of time five men were in the changing room. Some of the men there were going to go to Gantry number three, a pencil bean proton machine used to radiate specific areas beyond the prostate. This machine rotated around the patient and shot a small pencil beam of proton radiation as it did so. This approach allowed for better control of where the proton radiation was delivered. The rest of the men and I were to receive treatment in Gantry four used for treating encapsulated cancer confined to the prostate. One of the men described the number three proton bean as being like a dot matrix printer in that it shot a pencil thin ray of proton beam at specific areas with greater precision than the number four gantry which shot a broader beam at the entire prostate.

"Hot Flashes"

I quickly discovered that humor was the major activity in the patient changing area. One of the standing jokes was the reaction men on hormone therapy experienced from taking female hormones to shrink their prostate and the size of the cancer tumor prior to proton therapy. Prostate cancer growth is fueled by the male hormone, androgen, and female hormones stopped it cold. One of the popular jokes among men who were receiving hormone therapy was related to the hot flashes they experienced. Henry was on hormone therapy and told me that since being given female hormones he had developed an irresistible urge to go shopping. Another burst of laughter followed Henry's well-delivered joke. Some of the other men taking female hormones also complained about the side effects they were experiencing and they frequently joked about gaining weight and having their breasts get slightly larger. A common joke was their asking each other what was their bra size that day. As the men exaggerated the side effects of hormone therapy, it lessened their concern over why they had to take this additional therapy.

The Balloon!

But the biggest source of ongoing humor and the topic to be surely brought up several times each day was the balloon.

As I stood dressed in my double surgical gowns, one of the men who had just come in, and seeing it was my first day, looked at me with a mischievous grin on his face and said, "Do you know she is going stick a balloon up your butt?" He then laughed and was joined by the other men. One of them added, "That's the fun part."

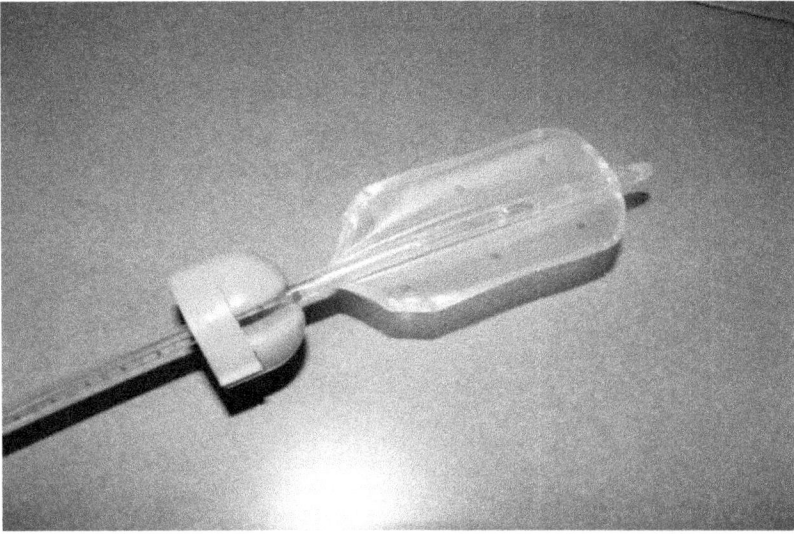

The Balloon

"Mr. Dawley, I'm ready for you," Sara said as she spotted me in the changing area.

Sara led me to a room next to the waiting room where she had me lie down.

Once inside the room, Sara handed me a towel and told me to cover my genitals and pull up my gown so she could scan my bladder with a hand held sonogram.

Sara asked for my card and told me that there were two numbers on the card that are very important. The first number was the bladder capacity I needed to have to ensure proper alignment of my prostate so that radiation would not go elsewhere. My targeted bladder capacity was between 300 and 370. The other number was the placing of my feet on the treatment gantry. My number for my feet placement was 60. These two measurements ensured my proper alignment when the beam was delivered.

After Sara scanned my bladder, she took a cup and drew a line near the top of it. Giving the cup to me she stated "Go to the restroom and urinate into this cup to fill it up to this line. Then empty the urine into the toilet, discard the cup, and walk down the hallway and enter another hallway across from this room.

After I followed her directions I returned to the hallway and walked into the treatment room. It was surrounded by a thick concrete wall designed, I imagined, for controlling the spread of radiation. It was also extremely well lit.

Cautiously walking in the treatment room, I saw Sara on the left by some monitors with a number of gauges. On my right I saw treatment gantry four, the machine that was going to deliver the life saving proton beam to me. It was huge.

I looked at the proton beam machine for a moment. It was a big machine that looked like it was hanging upside down. There were several devices that I later discovered were X-ray machines on both sides of the treatment table.

"Please take off your second gown, Mr. Dawley" Sara requested.

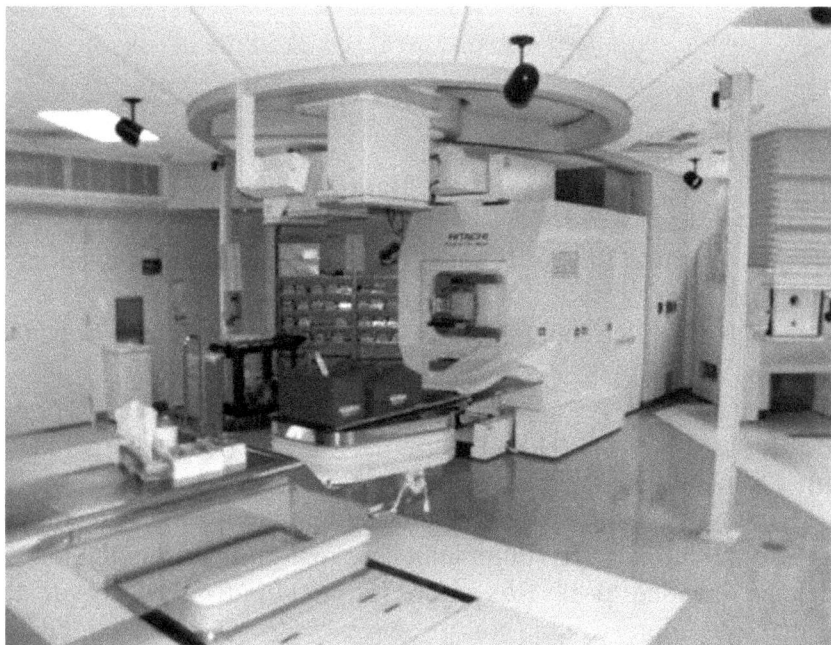

Proton Beam Gantry Number Four

Sara led me by the hand to the treatment platform directly in the front of the proton beam machine and told me to lie down on the table, raise my knees, and to cover my genital area with the towel.

Sara then approached and told me she was going to place some lubricant on my anus and would then insert a balloon into my rectum, adding, "I will then fill the balloon with water and it will keep your rectum away from the radiation that will be directed to your prostate. We will shoot the proton beam at your prostate from one side and will turn the platform around and will then shot it again from the other side. You don't have to do anything other than lie still."

Sara then handed me a large V shaped piece of plastic and told me to hold it in my hands,

With skillful ease Sara gently applied the lubricant to my anus and then slowly inserted the balloon device. It wasn't a bad experience.

Once she had the balloon in my rectum she said "I am now going to fill it with water and you will feel a sense of fullness."

Sara filled the balloon and just as she said I would I felt a sense of fullness like I had to have a bowel movement. Again, it felt a bit strange but was not an unpleasant experience.

Sara then went about adjusting the proton beam device and inserting some device into the front from where I later learned the beam would come. An opening shaped like my prostate had been cut in a brass plate and it would ensure that the beam radiated my prostate and went nowhere else.

Sara then took several x-rays. Then the platform was adjusted based on the coordinates of the markers inserted into my prostate and moved slightly up and to one side, Sara then checked the alignment of my body again to make doubly sure I was properly aligned.

The x-rays were done to ensure I was always properly aligned for treatment by using the fiducials that had been inserted into my bladder. One day Sara showed me an x-ray of the fiducials. She would first of all take an x-ray in which the fiducial markers would show up. Using these markers as guidelines she would then adjust the table so that I would be perfectly aligned to receive the proton beam into my prostate. During each of my treatment sessions my positioning was carefully checked to ensure I was perfectly aligned so the proton therapy radiation would hit the cancer cells and not harm surrounding healthy tissue.

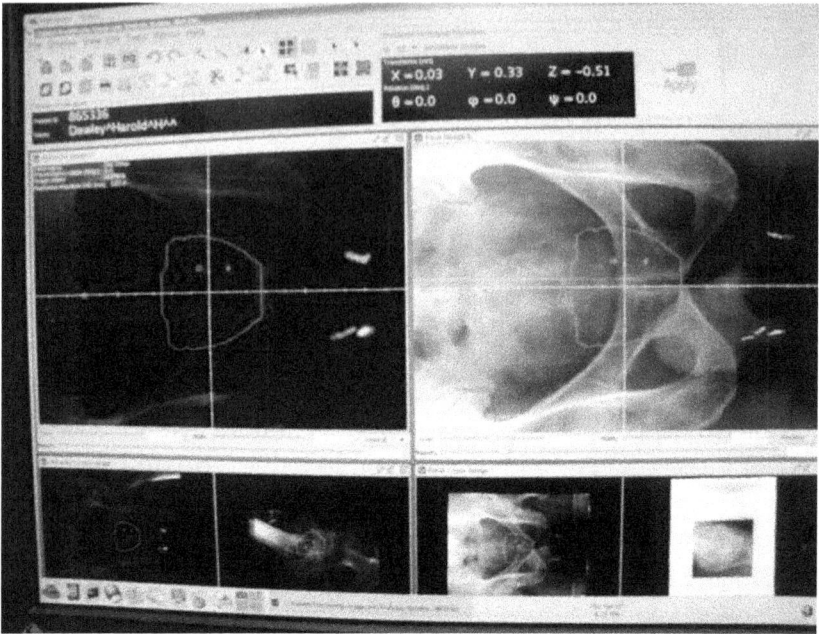

Fiducial markers are evident as the two dots in the enclosed area around my prostate.

Sara was wonderful. She explained to me what was going on and that the four treatment gantries all shared the same beam. A medical physicist and my physician had developed a treatment plan in which a certain amount of radiation would be directed through the aperture shaped like my prostate directly to my prostate.

"I will let you know when it is our turn for the beam," Sara stated.

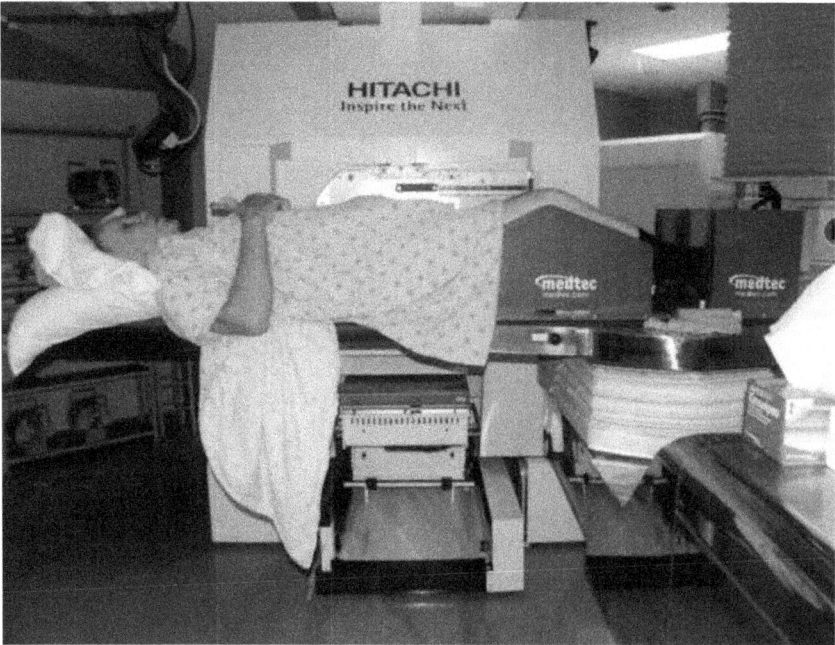

I lay on the treatment gantry four awaiting the beam.

"We've Got the Beam"

Sara was over by the control center on one side of the room when she turned to me and said what is undoubtedly the most important statement heard in proton therapy "We've got the beam."

A warning bell then went off as Sara retreated to a lead encased room. I heard some hissing noise and some slight rattling. Then a slightly higher pitch was heard for about eight seconds as the proton beam entered my prostate. That was it, short and sweet.

About 20 seconds later, Sara entered the room and worked the controls so that the platform on which I was lying was turned so that the proton beam could be directed to my prostate from a different angle.

Shortly later Sara again said, "We've got the beam."

After I received the second dose of proton radiation, Sara entered the room and brought the platform back down to a lower level. Sara approached and told me to raise my knees, adding, "I will now release the water from the balloon and then withdraw it from you."

I could feel the balloon shrink in size as water was released from it. Sara then began a slow withdrawal of the balloon. This was a truly strange experience; while not overly unpleasant, it always seemed like it took a lot longer to withdraw the balloon than it did inserting it. It was a relief when it was finally out.

"That's it Mr. Dawley, you are free to go."

"Was It Fun?"

Relieved that my first treat session was over, I quickly walked back to the patient changing area. I also had to urinate and my pace picked up. There were now around six men there awaiting their turn for treatment.

The men looked up and smiled at me as I quickly walked in and headed to the toilet.

"Was it fun?" one of the men asked as he and the others laughed good-naturedly.

"I can't say it was fun but I can tell you I'm glad to be done with my first treatment." I responded.

"Your only have 38 more to go," one of the men replied.

I urinated and felt the relief of no longer maintaining a seventy-five-percent- full bladder.

I opened my locker and changed into my street clothes. I then put the two gowns and the towel into a large hamper. When I stepped into the waiting room, I stood there listening to the ongoing conversation. The men were careful to involve me in their discussion and it was an enjoyable experience. That day was the last day for one of the men. As tradition dictated, he brought in some pastries for everyone. I stayed and ate a pastry, a nice big donut with diced sugarcoated apples. One of the men, an airline pilot, said he was going to bring some more donuts the following morning as it was his last day. It was a pleasant experience. I already felt like I was a member of that little informal group.

Upon leaving the treatment area, I walked down the hallway leading to the downstairs waiting room where I noticed several men gathered around an oriental looking gong of some sort suspended in the air by chains and hanging from a wooden support. I had seen this device before and wondered why it was there.

Pausing, I watched the scene that unfolded in front of me.

One man was holding the beater that was attached to the gong, and, facing the other three men around him, stated, "As is the tradition here I now beat this gong to symbolize my beating cancer." Having made that statement the man beat the gong while his friends clapped their hands.

Just then a man came up from behind, and, sensing I was new, stated, "It is a tradition that after you finish your treatment you beat this gong to symbolize beating cancer."

"Good idea," I replied.

Walking out that first morning I felt good about my decision to receive treatment at the proton therapy center. Every man I had talked to that first day had nothing but positive statements about the treatment and the treatment staff. Plus, I already felt accepted into the group of patients whose treatment time was around mine and that really made me feel good.

Walking out into the crowded waiting area, I saw Linda sitting down talking with several couples. When I joined her, she introduced me to the people with whom she was talking. *More friendly people*, I thought to myself, as I joined the discussion.

Finally, as we drove back to our apartment, I told Linda how glad I was that I had decided to get the proton beam treatment at MD Anderson.

Linda agreed and stated she felt the same way.

As I lay in bed that night I thought about how a bond was forming with the men going through treatment much like a bond that forms among men in combat. Having spent the bulk of my career in psychology evaluating and treating veterans, many of whom saw combat, the analogy of combat frequently came to my mind. Suddenly I realized that those of us going through treatment together were warriors in the war on cancer. Just as troops in combat bond together and draw strength for one another, those of us going through treatment together were bonding together. A flash of inspiration hit me as I decided to write a book on my treatment experience with the title "Proton Warriors." The next morning I ordered a large banner stating "Proton Warriors" and when it arrived shortly thereafter I tacked it up on the wall of the patient changing. You will see it in a number of the photos in this book. The last time I checked, it was still on the wall and overflowing with signatures of men going through proton therapy. If you go to the proton therapy center, go ahead and sign your name on it.

Chapter Seven

The Social Aspects of Treatment

Together we stand, divided we fall

The Warrior Bond

Those of us who are diagnosed with cancer know well the fear of death. Just the word cancer conjures up anxiety in most people. When we're told we have cancer it is virtually always accompanied by fear. Prostate cancer can kill us and it is the third leading cause of death for men so it is not something to be taken lightly. Fear of this magnitude is also common among men facing the threat of death in combat, and is commonly experienced in war. There are similarities between fighting for our lives in the war on cancer and fighting as part of a military unit in the combat of war. This Chapter points out some of these similarities and my experience in going through treatment with a group of men with whom I became friends.

Let's begin with the importance that intimidation can play on our level of fear. In military combat, opposing sides frequently try to intimidate their enemy to weaken their will to fight. In the late 1800's, British troops wore a large bearskin cap that was over a foot tall. When their enemies looked across the battlefield they would see British soldiers that looked to be six to seven feet tall and such a sight had an intimidating effect. Some of the enemy would lose their will to fight and give up before the battle even began. A similar reaction can occur in some of us when we discover we have cancer and we become intimidated by fear and, for some of us, our will to fight can be weakened. This is not good.

Espirit de Corps

Long ago, humans learned that it was easier to face danger and the threat of death while in the company of people they trusted and to whom they felt close. Fear was not as intense when they had trusted friends and comrades standing beside them than when they stood alone. The history of warfare is replete with examples of military units who fought bravely and effectively against superior odds by bonding together in tight, cohesive units. The strong bond evident in such units is frequently referred to as Espirit de Corps and the stronger it is the braver the units fought.

There's an interesting event that occurred in the last year of WWII in the European campaign that relates to combat fatigue and the presence or absence of close ties. American troops began experiencing a high rate of combat fatigue that alarmed the Allied High Command. As more and more soldiers developed combat fatigue, the Americans looked at the German units facing them and discovered that they had a significantly lower rate of combat fatigue. When they looked more closely at how the German units operated they saw that whenever their units reached a certain level of casualties they were pulled out of combat and sent to the rear and replacements were added. The units then trained together until the new men were assimilated into the unit and established close bonds with the other soldiers. Once the unit formed a tight cohesive bond they were sent back to combat.

The American policy was to simply send in new replacements, as casualties were experienced. Soon units lost their cohesiveness as new men replaced those killed or wounded. Soldiers found themselves facing the threat of death with other men they did not know and with whom they had not established a close, supportive relationship. In such a situation the fear of death became so great the men suffered combat fatigue.

The Americans quickly adopted the German policy of pulling units out of combat when they reached a certain level of casualties and sending in replacements who trained with them until the unit once again formed into a strong supportive group. After they made this change, the rate of combat fatigue dropped dramatically to that of the Germans.

In health care the presence of strong, supportive bonds with other people is identified as social support and it's just as important in fighting threats to our health as in facing threats in war. Combat units with good camaraderie or possessing Esprit de corps do well. Likewise, numerous studies have clearly demonstrated the importance of social support in dealing with heart disease, cancer, and many other illnesses. The better our relations are with the people in our life such as spouse, parents, children, other relatives, and friends, the better are our odds in dealing with health threats.

Social Support

The odds of successfully fighting threats go way down for those who lack supportive social relationships referred to as social support. During my tenure as a staff psychologist at the New Orleans Veterans Affairs Medical Center, I observed the valuable role social support can play in health care. For a number of years I was assigned to several medical/surgical wards and my job was to answer consultation requests from physicians who were concerned about the mental or emotional status of their patients. Generally, such concerns arose from the physician's perception that the patient was depressed or suffered from some other type of emotional distress. In answering these consults, I began to notice a major difference between patients assigned to a separate room and those who were placed in a large bay or dormitory setting shared with many other veterans.

I quickly discovered that I had many more consults on men who were assigned to a single room. I would typically arrive at the single rooms to find the veteran lying down with an obvious appearance of being depressed. In talking with them their affect was flat and they exhibited all of the symptoms of depression. I discovered that many of them did not have much social support. They were widowed, divorced, or separated, and had little contact with family members. Most of these men had little opportunity to meet and mingle with other patients and many stayed isolated in their room. In contrast most veterans assigned to large dormitory settings were not depressed. They had a more optimistic attitude as they interacted together and got to know each other. I would frequently walk into one of these large bays and see groups of veterans sitting on each others' beds engaged in animated conversations. Everyone seemed to know one another and a sense of unity was evident. In short, the veterans in the dormitory setting had a chance to develop supportive relationships with their fellow veterans while those in single rooms didn't. It made a big difference to their emotional health.

Shortly before I retired from the New Orleans Veterans Affairs Medical Center, it was in the process of eliminating the large dormitory settings and moving all patients to single rooms. *What a mistake*, I thought, as I observed this unfortunate policy unfold.

So, how does combat in WWII and whether or not a veteran is assigned to a single bedroom or to a dormitory with many other veterans present relate to your being treated for prostate cancer?

It all relates to the remarkable power of bonding, the social support it provides, and the important role bonding with fellow prostate cancer patients plays in treating our cancer.

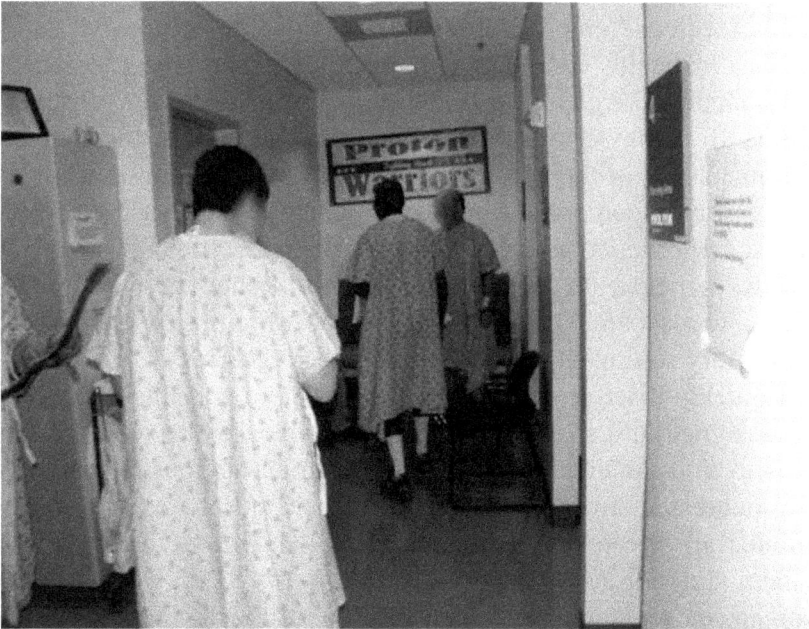

Proton pals laughing and joking together as part of their daily treatment routine.

Social Bonding – The Unexpected Bonus of Proton Therapy

"Yeah, when I got the call from my urologist that I had prostate cancer I was flabbergasted," Rex (a pseudonym) told me as we relaxed together in comfortable chairs in one of the patient changing rooms at the Proton Therapy Center, adding "I just didn't think I had cancer."

For the previous five days, Rex and I had generally arrived at the same time. We were usually the first to arrive. After we changed into our gowns, we sat down and socialized with each other.

"I felt the same way when I got my phone call from my doctor telling me I had cancer," I replied.

Rex continued "My doctor told me he would go over it in more detail when we met. I told him I could come in right away since I wanted to know what I was facing but he replied I would have to call his office and schedule an appointment. I had to wait three days before I could see him! It was three days of hell."

I replied that when my doctor called and told me I had cancer he took his time and made sure I fully understood everything he was saying. I added that he kept asking me if I understood and did I have any further questions. I stated that I felt he was genuinely emphatic and concerned for me.

"Not mine," Rex replied adding that his doctor seemed more concerned about "my letting him do the surgery on me than encouraging me to look around for what I thought was the best treatment option."

"I got his call telling me I had cancer on a Friday and I spent the weekend doing research on the Internet on the various ways to treat prostate cancer. I saw a lot of advertisements and articles encouraging men with prostate cancer to try specific treatments but as I continued reading I saw that many of them had bad side effects. It seemed to me that surgery and conventional radiation therapy resulted in a high incidence of urinary incontinence and loss of sexual functioning. There were other articles or reports of 'new' treatments such as when they freeze the cancer but on reading further I saw that they also had the same bad side effects. Then I started seeing something unique – actual reports by patients who went through proton beam therapy describing the benefits of this treatment. After reading a number of such reports I went to the MD Anderson website and read about its Proton Therapy Center's treatment program for prostate cancer. The more I read the better it looked," Rex stated.

"I more or less did the same thing," I replied.

"When I finally saw my doctor, he tried really hard to get me do surgery with him. But I had made up my mind and had, in fact, already signed up for the Proton Therapy center prostate treatment program," Rex added.

"Now that I am about two-thirds through treatment, I am very happy I selected this method. Many of the guys I work with are asking me about it as several have prostate cancer. I'm now like the guys I saw on the Internet extolling the benefits of proton therapy. It works!"

As Rex and I sat in the patient changing area talking with each other, I thought to myself about the bond of friendship that was developing between us. I enjoyed talking with Rex and the other men and much of my fear of the unexpected melted away as I did so.

Just then Henry, the resident comedian walked in and cheerfully said hello.

"I got hit with hot flashes last night and when I turned down the AC, my girlfriend said I was a wimp because women going through the change of life handle them without freezing to death the people around them," Henry stated bringing laughs from us.

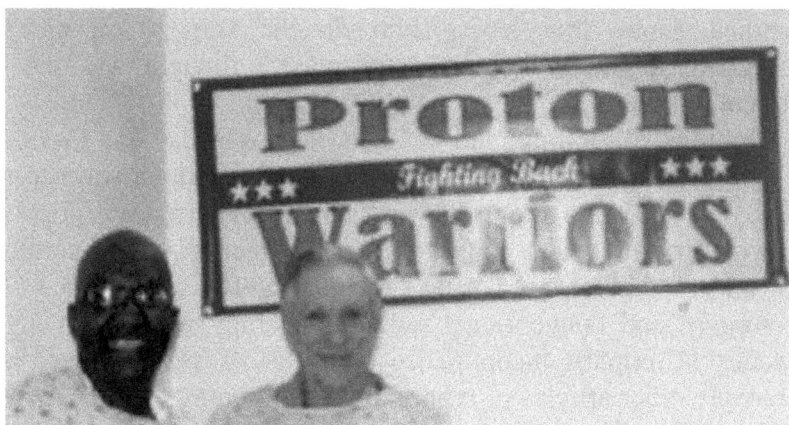

Henry the comedian and Author

Several additional patients soon entered and a buzz of conversation started. Now that Henry had a bigger audience his comedic charm kicked into full swing.

"I was driving home yesterday when I passed this shopping center and had this irresistible urge to stop and buy a pair of shoes," Henry delivered skillfully with a deadpan expression and an apparent sense of genuine concern.

Loud laughter followed Henry's humor.

Jim, one of the patients nearing the end of his treatment arrived next and announced that he and his wife were inviting everyone to their beachfront home on Wednesday for a celebration party.

Just then several of the patients burst out in laughter as Carl came shuffling in as fast as he could, carefully covering his exposed backside.

"I gotta go, gotta go, make way, make way," Carl called out as he made a beeline for the bathroom.

Then the unexpected happened. Since it is very important to keep our bladder at a certain capacity and some of the men had difficulty holding it, accidents occasionally happened. The treatment staff had the solution to this problem by providing those who had difficulty holding their urine with a small latching device they were to put over their penis whenever they felt they couldn't hold their urine any longer but their treatment was not complete. At that point they were to put this device over their penis and clap it shut. The clap was lined with a spongy material so it was not hard when placed around the penis and it worked.

Unknown to us, Carl had put one of these devices on his penis even though he had never used it before. Once in the toilet Carl started cursing up a storm. He then yelled out "HELP, HELP, I can't get this damn thing off me – call a technician I need help now." One of the guys standing near the hallway yelled down to the technician on duty, that he was needed, "right now!"

Carl's yelling increased and he was obviously in pain. The technician came running quickly and entering the toilet saw that Carl was tightening the clamp instead of loosening it.

The technician promptly undid the clamp and Carl let out a loud sign of relief as his strong stream of urine was released into the toilet bowl.

For a good week, Carl's story was told, re-told and embellished, as the patients came and left for their treatments. Even though his story grew a bit, Carl was a good sport and joined the laughter whenever it was told to someone who had not heard it. This experience helped to draw everyone together.

Social Outings and Other Events

Captivated by the warm feeling of camaraderie growing in me for my friends, I announced one morning that my wife and I were having a wine and cheese party at our apartment that coming Sunday from 2 to 4 PM. I encouraged all of the patients present in the patient changing area to attend. I then placed a sheet announcing our party on the door of the bathroom - the spot where every patient made at least two trips on every visit.

That Sunday, we had our first party.

During our wine and cheese party I sat enjoying the warm friendship of my friends and laughed with them at their jokes and sometimes off-colored humor. Sitting there I found myself thinking about how unique and unexpected was the degree of social bonding that was occurring as we all went through treatment together. Dumfounded, I realized that I was not even thinking about being treated for prostate cancer but was instead having fun being with our new friends.

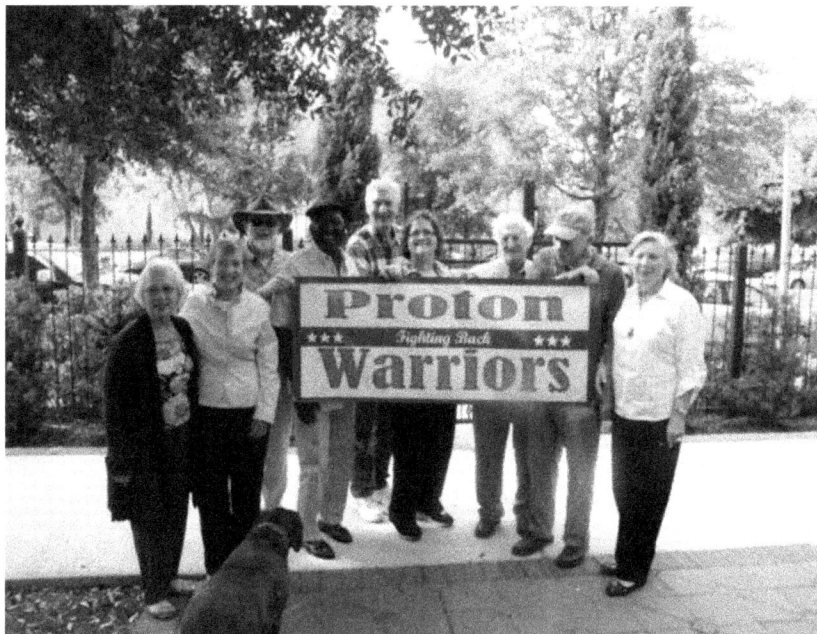

Lina, Judy, Bob, Henry, Steve, Marcia, Joe, Harold, & Linda - Proton pals enjoying a wine and cheese party. (Dog is Susie – owned by someone else having a party at same time)

One of the really nice aspects of going through the Proton Therapy Center program are the weekly dinners in which 15 to 25 patients and their wives - or their significant others- gather at different restaurants. At the MD Anderson Proton Therapy Center these are generally arranged by ProtonPals, a patient support organization led by Joe Landry, who had gone through the proton therapy center years earlier. A patient who volunteered to do so would run the dinners and sometimes a staff member would join the group. Dinner arrangements were made at one of five or six restaurants near the proton therapy center that have a separate room or dining area to accommodate such a large group. Starting around 5:30 PM, the event begins with a cocktail hour where we have wine or other alcoholic drinks or soft drinks and meet and mingle with one another.

These dinners are a good way of meeting other patients who are receiving their treatment at different times. On my first dinner meeting I was introduced as a new patient and was immediately welcomed by several people who came over and shook my hand and welcomed me aboard. One especially pleasant woman took me by the hand and told my wife and me that we were going to sit with her and her husband. It was only after we were seated with them that I discovered that her husband was a retired Air Force two star general. As a Marine Corps veteran who only made it to E-3 in my three year enlistment, the third lowest enlisted rank, sitting next to a retired two star general, the third highest obtainable officer rank, was quite an experience for me. In the Marines, senior enlisted non-commissioned officers such as 1ST Sergeants and Sergeant Majors are held in high esteem. But a general, a two star general in particular, is like a deity. The general brushed my awe aside by stating luck was a large part of achieving the rank of general. He and his wife were delightful. I was sorry that he graduated a week later.

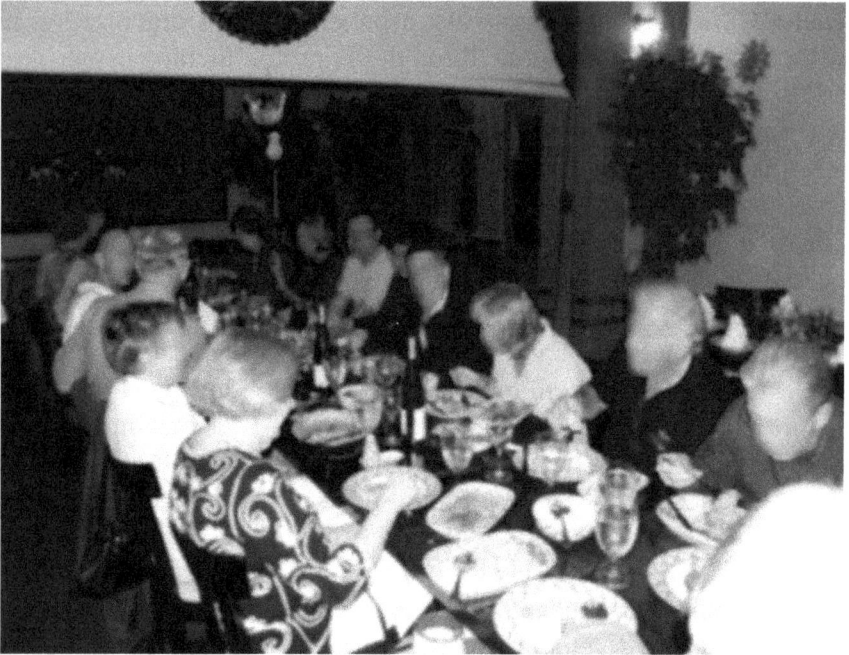

Proton pals enjoying another weekly eat out together.

Everyone is friendly at the social gatherings. After one or two before dinner drinks a buzz of conversation develops as we all interact together. A dinner coordinator is selected for every batch of patients going through the proton therapy. A pleasant real estate broker in his late forties or early fifties was the coordinator when I went through. Another patient, a landscaper in his early fifties, assisted him. Both were very outgoing and naturally comfortable with people. Each had an attractive wife, and their contributions made the dinners a very positive and enjoyable activity to which we all looked forward. For my last two weeks I was the coordinator. At the last dinner I transferred the responsibility for coordinating the dinners to another patient who had volunteered to do it. For several of the dinners Joe Landry, the founder of Protonpals.net was present. Tai Lee, a Vietnamese-American nurse practitioner staff member that we all loved would sometimes join us at the dinners.

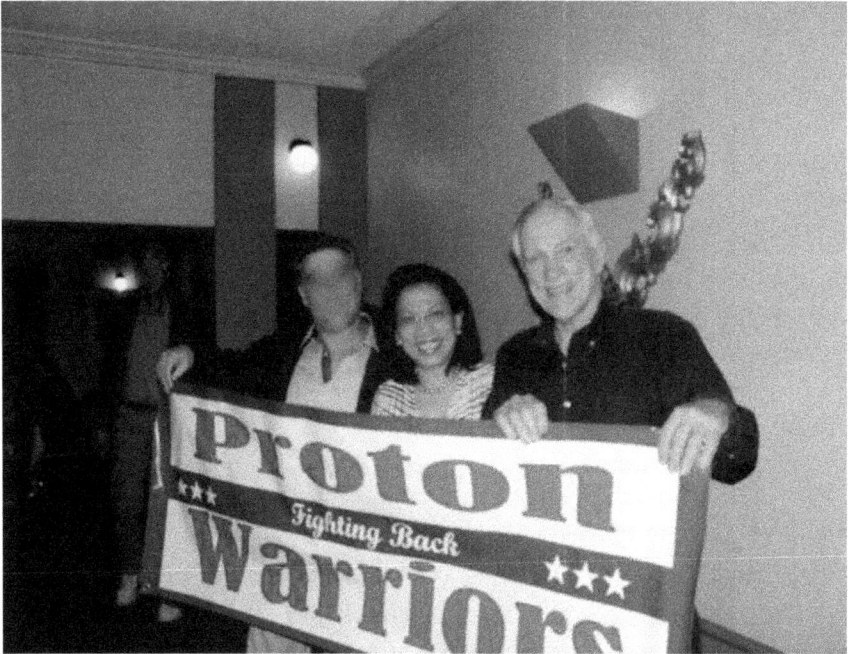

Tai Lee and Author

Other spontaneous smaller social events developed among the patients as we got to know one another. In our case we had several wine and cheese parties attended by Henry the comedian and six other patients with their spouses. We also went to see the movie *The King's Speech* with three other couples and then had dinner afterwards. We also went to a couple of nice restaurants with several other couples on a number of other occasions. On each occasion we invariably reverted to the bawdy humor from our patient changing area and ended up laughing so hard our sides would hurt. Plus there was a delightful day in which we went to a gulf front beach home of one of the patients who had just graduated, and spent a wonderful time socializing together amid good food and drinks. I remember standing on his Gulf front home and watching the sunset feeling amazed at how my treatment experience was so pleasant. We all looked like pictures of good health. No one was in pain or discomfort. In fact, at times we had to remind ourselves we were not on vacation but instead were fighting cancer.

Prior to starting my treatment, a staff member had casually suggested we get an apartment close to Herman Park and enjoy the sites in Houston. We followed that advice and to our pleasant surprise my treatment at the proton therapy center and our stay at that apartment was indeed more like a vacation, one of our better vacations at that!

Whenever Linda and I would see or talk with some of our friends back home, they would express solemn concern over how I was doing since I was a cancer patient. We would then excitedly tell them about all of the fun we were having. One friend even sent us an e-mail admonishing us to "tone it down a bit." Our friends could not believe we were having so much fun. My treatment experience was a strange yet rewarding period in which my wife and I got close to many of the other patients. It was an active period with just about every week bringing three or more social outings. It was in many ways a very enjoyable experience.

What is Social Bonding?

Social bonding refers to establishing positive, satisfying, and enjoyable relationships with other people. Such relationships happen naturally in all facets of our lives. They generally occur quicker and in a more satisfying manner when two ingredients are present: propinquity and proximity. Add a common cause and the threat of danger and all the ingredients are there for strong bonding.

Proximity and Propinquity: It was while I was writing the book *Friendship – How To Make And Keep Friends*[1] published by Prentice Hall a number of years ago, that I first became aware of the importance of proximity and propinquity are in the formation of friendships.

Proximity refers to your nearness or physical closeness to another person or people and how often you are close to them. An example of being in close proximity with someone would be your next-door neighbors. The reality is that you are physically close to these neighbors on an ongoing basis. This close proximity can increase the likelihood of a friendly relationship developing just as the sheer distance from someone living on the other side of town that you seldom see decreases the likelihood of a relationship developing.

Propinquity is slightly different from proximity in that it refers to the increased opportunity for interaction. A good example is your job. You likely have close proximity with a number of fellow workers but if there is nothing that compels you to interact with them there is less likelihood of a warm, supportive relationship. But if you work in a special section consisting of five people with whom you have to interact closely in the sense of asking and answering questions, solving problems together, and pursuing common goals, the chances are good that friendships will develop. Not all people who work closely together with fellow workers develop positive relationships and some may even develop negative relationships. The chances are, however, greater that a positive relationship will develop when propinquity is also present.

And that brings us to the proton therapy.

Some of our closest relationships are established when we are in close proximity with others with whom we are pursuing the same goal or facing a common threat. This is why some of our best friendships are developed in school and college or in the military and similar settings in which we are in close proximity with other people involved in similar activities such as training together or pursuing a degree. The social bond becomes even stronger when an element of danger or threat is present. As a Veterans Affairs psychologist I saw the incredibly strong bonds that developed among veterans who served in combat together. It is for this reason that veterans' organizations have always existed for as long as wars have been fought. The Grand Army of the Republic flourished after the Civil War as Union veterans joined to be with their fellow union veterans. Several years later in 1889 the United Confederate Veterans Association was formed. After World War I, the Veterans of Foreign Wars and American Legion formed. After WWII, AMVETS was formed and later, the Vietnam Veterans of America. More recently, the Iraq and Afghanistan Veterans of America was formed as these veterans also sought the company of their fellow veterans.

A similar bond develops among men going through the proton center treatment for their prostate cancer. They, too, find themselves in close proximity with each other as they spend eight weeks going through proton therapy treatment together facing their common threat of prostate cancer and becoming friends.

The Brotherhood of the Balloon – Robert Marckini

The Brotherhood of the Balloon is an organization for patients who are going through or who have gone through proton therapy treatment in California at Loma Linda Medical Center. Robert Marckini founded it after he successfully completed proton therapy at the Loma Linda Medical Center for the treatment of his prostate cancer. Bob went on to write the excellent book YOU CAN BEAT PROSTATE CANCER AND YOU DON'T NEED SURGERY TO DO IT.[2] Bob also has an excellent website ProtonBob.com where a wealth of information is available describing prostate cancer, proton beam therapy, along with testimonials from patients who beat their prostate cancer by going through proton therapy. His book is undoubtedly the best book ever written about proton therapy and is a must reading for anyone considering it. Accessing Bob's wonderful site and reading the testimonials on it helped me to select proton beam therapy for my prostate cancer. According to Bob's website, ProtonBob.com, the Brotherhood of the Balloon now has over 5000 members (and their families) that belong to the organization. In the history of proton beam treatment of prostate cancer, Bob stands out as an important contributor to the growth and increasing popularity of this effective treatment.

Proton Pals – Joe Landry

While Brotherhood of the Balloon represents men who have gone through treatment at the Loma Linda Medical Center, Protonpals.net is another organization that has been formed by Joe Landry for patients who have completed treatment or are undergoing treatment in Houston at MD Anderson's Proton Therapy Center. A Ph.D. chemical engineer, Joe was also impressed by the pioneering efforts of Bob Marckini in establishing The Brotherhood of the Balloon and saw the need for a similar organization for patients who were going through the MD Anderson Proton Therapy Center in Houston. Shortly thereafter Joe established Protonpals.net. It is now a vibrant organization with a newsletter that goes out to a large number of patients who have gone through the proton therapy center for their prostate cancer. Joe is still actively involved with patients going through Proton Therapy. I had the pleasure of meeting Joe and getting to know him and his lovely wife Marcia, and becoming good friends with them.

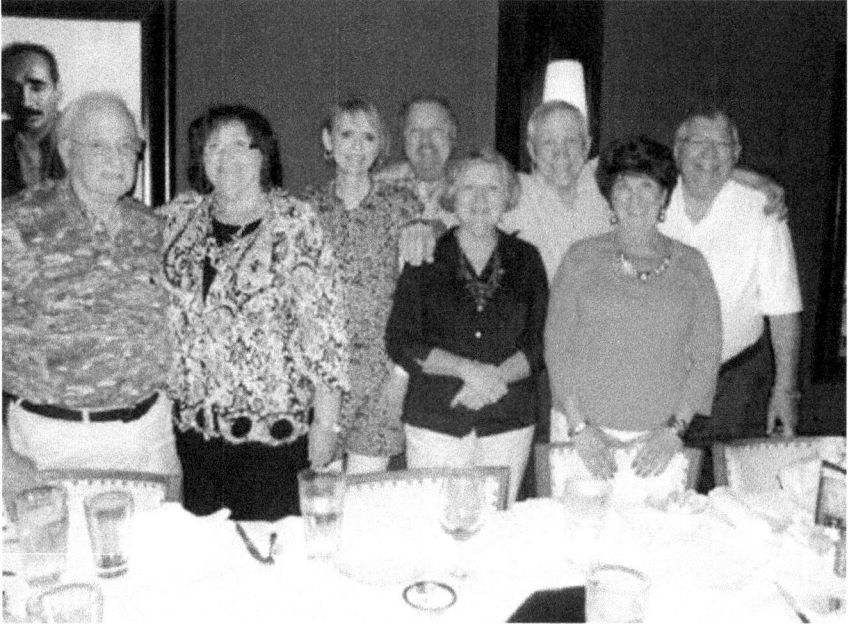

Left to right - Joe, Marcia, Cindy, Tom, Linda, Harold, Pam, and Gary.

The Benefits of Facing Threat Together

As I progressed through proton therapy for my prostate cancer, I looked forward each day to interacting with the friends I had developed. While no one can be a friend with everyone and sometimes for whatever reason, we just don't click with someone, I can't recall anyone I encountered during my treatment with whom I was not able to develop a positive and supportive relationship. The unique circumstances of the situation in which we found ourselves made developing such bonds a highly likely event. Like a squad of men in combat covering each other's back evolving into a closely knit warrior bond, in going through treatment together to save our lives from the threat of cancer we became a tight, cohesive group.

Saying Goodbye to Warrior Friends and Welcoming New Ones

The daily routine of laughing, sometimes uncontrollably about balloons being inserted in us and holding our urine till it hurt built strong bonds of friendship among us as we went through treatment.

But when I reached my sixth week of treatment, something strange happened that made me realize the strength of this bond.

Let me first of all state that there were a few times when I had the first treatment appointments in the morning in which I would arrive early and no one else was present. On these occasions I found myself sitting alone in the patient changing area and soon a strange, different feeling came over me. As I sat there, alone, I found myself staring at the empty chairs and blank walls and began to feel lonely. This feeling was followed by a sense of insecurity and a vague sense of threat. I yearned for the companionship of my friends and without it I felt insecure and vulnerable. Fortunately, these moments were few as other men soon joined me and I reestablished my social bonds.

But as I neared the end of my treatment another vague sense of loss and unhappiness slowly began to grow. I was so pleased and happy with the social bonding that any inhibitions I had were quickly dissipated and I was a good second to Henry's comic act. We would play off each other like a comedy act. He did, however, steal some of my jokes but in a spirit of camaraderie, I forgave him. We were, after all, a good comedic team. I would either bear the brunt of one of his jokes or would help his joke come off well by saying or acting in certain ways. But one day Henry completed his treatment with two other friends. As the men stood next to the gong wearing silly looking balloons wrapped around their heads prepared by one of their wives, each made a moving farewell speech, Henry, as usual, used the occasion to do a comic routine centering on other balloons and where such balloons "will never go again," I joined in by asking him to bend over "once more for old time's sake." But that night and the following two days a vague sense of unhappiness and insecurity began growing inside me.

Strangely, my attitude toward coming to the proton therapy center changed. Instead of bouncing in with a big grin and a look of confidence, I quietly walked in feeling somewhat self-conscious. It was an unpleasant period; the only one I experienced during my treatment. Then I realized what was happening; I was going through a sense of loss as Henry and my other friends left the treatment program. This sense of loss in turn led to feelings of insecurity and vulnerability, as I felt alone.

"I feel awkward saying this," I said to Ray (a pseudonym), a man much younger but in many ways wiser than me, "as the men who have become my friends leave, I feel a sense of loss and sadness. I miss them and it also…. makes me feel somewhat insecure…."

Self-disclosure, the ability to reveal true inner feelings is a part of the friendship process as it allows people to see us as we really are.

"I know exactly how you feel, Ray replied. "I miss the guys I've gotten to know and to whom I got close and it also makes me sad and a bit insecure, too."

I immediately felt better hearing Ray shared the same feelings I was experiencing. The sense of loss and resultant feelings of insecurity we both felt came from the loss of our friends completing treatment and leaving. Once I realized what was going on I knew the antidote was to turn to the new friends among those going through treatment behind me. In other words, the old adage "don't look back, look forward" made sense as a way to deal with what Ray and I were experiencing. So for those of you, who go through proton therapy, be prepared for this experience to happen to you.

Just as I had established friendships with the men that were in the program when I arrived, other men who subsequently arrived also became my friends. Plus, I was enjoying their friendship just as much as I enjoyed the friendship of the men who had moved on. From that point on, I focused on my friends who were in the program even going as far as kidding them by saying, "Don't cry when I leave – because I know you're going to miss me."

SO HERE IT IS. Be prepared for a sense of loss as you get near the end of your treatment. Keep in mind it is normal. Draw camaraderie and support from the new men who are going through treatment behind you.

Chapter Eight

Completing Treatment

One of the happiest days in my life!

The Treatment Routine

The treatment routine was the same every day. I would begin by spending time with four to six other men receiving treatment in either Gantry 3 or Gantry 4 as we shared the same waiting/changing room. This was always an enjoyable experience as we joked and poked good-natured humor at each other.

Treatment was Monday through Friday for eight weeks. Linda and I would stay in Houston for two weeks and then my treatment technician, either Shane or Sara, would find another patient who was willing to swap my Monday 6:30 AM appointment for their late Monday evening appointment. This arrangement allowed us to spend three nights at our home in Diamondhead, MS, a six-hour drive from Houston every other weekend.

Humor remained the dominant theme during my eight weeks of treatment at the Proton Therapy Center. Several standard jokes were a routine part of every treatment session. As we sat together awaiting treatment we all shared the same concerns of not having enough urine in our bladder. Whenever one of us did not have enough urine in our bladder, we would lose our turn and then have to drink more water to reach our targeted level. Another cause of concern was gas. Not only was there a pronounced reluctance to pass gas whenever the technician, usually Sara or some other attractive young woman, inserted the balloon, as it would be embarrassing, but the presence of gas could also result in the proton beam being misaligned and hitting healthy, non-cancerous tissue. One of the patients, Henry, always carried a number of gas-x pills to minimize the danger of having gas and freely offered them to the rest of us. Keeping a full bladder was another ongoing concern. The sight of one of us rushing back to release some urine generally triggered laughter and jokes while going back and losing our turn because our level of urine was too low also generated more good-natured humor.

Graduations

Since new patients are continually being added and existing patients eventually complete their treatments, just about every day or so someone is completing treatment. The usual procedure is for that person to bring some treats for his fellow patients. This usually involves bringing in delicious treats such as large chocolate chip cookies or oversized oatmeal cookies that I just love. The word goes out for all patients and staff to help themselves to the treats. Sometimes the men brought a regular type bread that either contains sausage or jelly, a treat that did not tempt me. But the nice big, soft and sweet donuts and cookies are a different story. And that relates to a problem I encountered in my third week.

The Problem of Weight Gain

By my third week I had been to eight to ten graduations and had helped myself to a large number of delicious cookies and pastries. I didn't pay any heed to Linda's concern about the importance of maintaining my weight. I was, after all, a cancer patient and was thus entitled to treats. But when I weighed in at my third weekly meeting with my oncologist, Dr. Brown, her nurse, Carla, weighed me and saw that I had gained four pounds. I realized I was in trouble.

"Mr. Dawley," Carla began, "are you eating cookies and donuts at the graduation celebrations?"

"Yes," I replied guilty.

Carla continued, "You have gained four pounds and if you gain one more pound we are going to have to repeat your simulation, and you know what that means."

The image of another machine going into my rectum filled my mind and I quickly replied that I would lose weight.

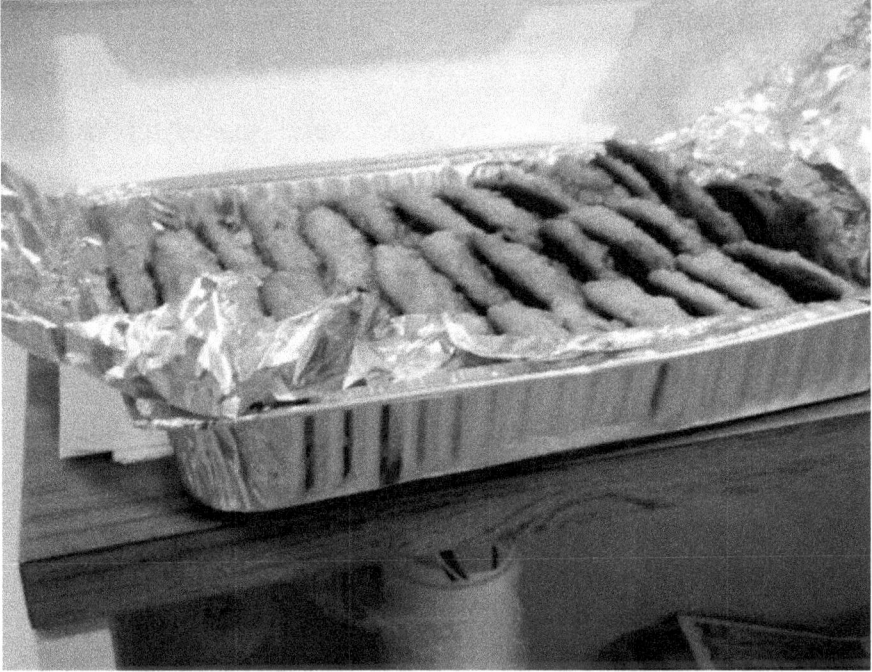

Delicious chocolate chip and oatmeal cookies provided by a man who graduated that day.

"The guys who finish their treatment want to share their happiness by bringing in donuts, cookies, and other treats. The problem is that they are very fattening and a number of our patients are gaining weight," Carla added.

"It is even a problem for us, the treatment staff," Carla continued. "They are so happy at finishing their treatment that they bring cookies, donuts, cakes and so forth up to us. We try not to eat them but when they are sitting in front of us all day it is hard not to do so. The average staff member gains 20 pounds their first year as a result of eating all of the sweets the patients bring to us when they graduate."

WARNING – Don't eat the sweets, or go lightly. Fresh fruit is OK.

The graduations are a fun experience. After meeting with the same group of guys on a daily basis for a number of weeks, you get to know them. There is almost continuous joking going on about different facets of the treatment with the leading joke being the balloon and the experience of it either going in or coming out (some dislike one more than the other). One man stated as part of his graduation address from "henceforth, my rectum will be a one way operation of my releasing material – nothing more will be accepted." His joke went over well.

Graduation is a big event to which we all looked forward. The man graduating brings in treats and then makes a short speech before hitting the oriental gong. Most of the men who are in his time slot usually attend the celebration along with his technician. The graduating patient's wife and family are usually present along with several other members of his treatment team. He makes a speech telling his friends goodbye and thanks the treatment staff. He then hits the gong. It's a nice experience.

We then go back to the patient changing area and usually bring two or three big, soft, and delicious chocolate chip cookies with us and await our turn for treatment.

My Treatment Went Fast

With scheduled weekly dinners at restaurants near the Proton Therapy Center and other impromptu social events time went by fast. I must admit that I did look forward to finishing my treatment and resuming my life. When my time to graduate drew near, I began to realize that I would miss many of the friends that I had made. In our last couple of weeks Linda and I made it a point to socialize with as many of our friends as we could.

My Graduation

We all experienced a bit of sadness as our friends graduated but we also knew that it was the beginning of a new life for them, one in which they would be cancer survivors. As my graduation date approached, I had progressed well in writing this book. One day Linda asked me if I wanted her to find a warrior costume that I could wear to my graduation ceremony. "Are you crazy, I'm not going to wear some silly costume," I self-righteously shot back and forgot about the idea. A week later Linda told me she had a surprise for me. She then pulled out a warrior's costume and suggested I wear it when I graduated from treatment. This time I didn't say anything but told myself I wouldn't have the nerve to wear it.

One night as we ate dinner with our friends in a pleasant side room in a good seafood restaurant in Houston, I told the five men and their spouses sitting around the table that, if I could work up the courage, I was going to wear a warrior's costume when I graduated.

"Go for it, Harold," Tom quickly responded.

"I think it is a great idea. It should get a laugh - which is always appreciated at the Proton Therapy Center," Gary added.

I had two weeks to go and I spent those two weeks debating if I had the nerve to wear the warrior's costume. I was beginning to warm to the idea of actually dressing up like a warrior. I would, in fact, be the "original proton warrior." I finally decided to wear the warrior's costume to my graduation but still had doubts if I had the courage to do so.

On my graduation day, still plagued by doubts, I tucked my costume in my bag and headed to the proton therapy center. I quickly entered the patient's changing area carrying my bag and pulled the curtain behind me. I hesitated briefly in the small changing booth and then put on the costume. I stood there looking at myself in the full-length mirror on the wall not believing what I was seeing.

I could hear my friends talking and joking out in the patient waiting area as I stood in the changing booth. I momentarily hesitated as my heart raced in a mixture of fear and excitement. *What if no one says anything and they just ignore me?* I agonized. I finally picked up the cheap plastic shield Linda made and the small plastic sword she found and insisted on my using with my costume and again stared at myself in the full-length mirror. *I don't believe it*, I thought to myself. Swallowing hard with my heart beating fast, I reached up and jerked the curtain open and quickly stepped outside of the booth. There I stood wearing a silly looking warrior costume holding a shield in my left hand and brandishing the plastic sword in the other as I faced the six other men in the waiting room. All conversation suddenly stopped as I stood there facing the other men for a few moments, which seemed like an eternity. They looked at me with dumfounded expressions on their faces as my heart raced even more. After a few seconds they burst out in laughter. I immediately felt relaxed and was glad I had let Linda talk me into wearing the costume.

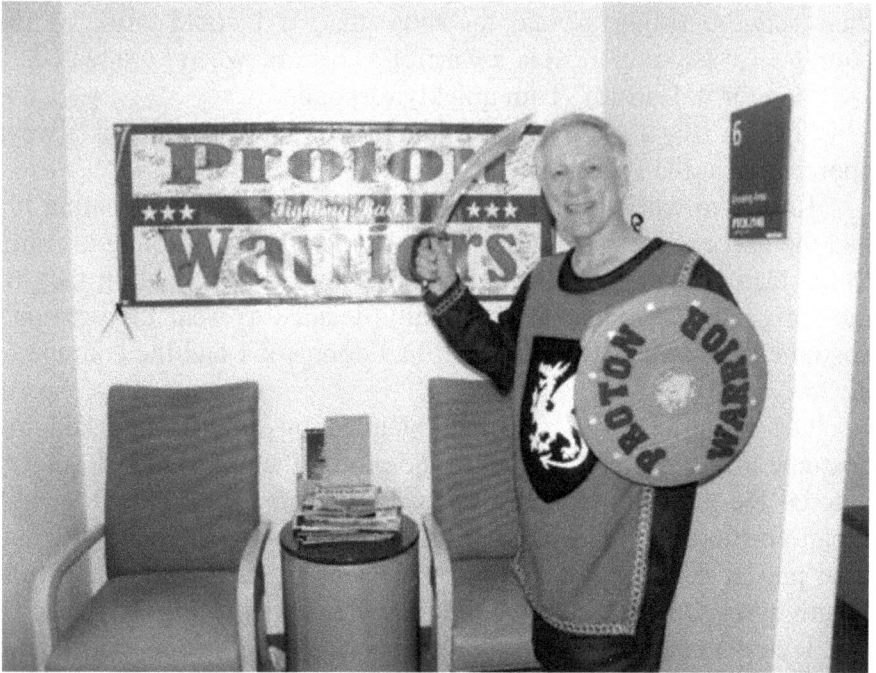

The "original proton warrior" in full military attire

I felt so good that I walked out into the hallway where passing staff looked at me in disbelief. I could see them wondering what that old man with the bird legs was doing wearing a warrior's costume. I brandished my sword at them until they laughed.

When Sara came to get me to do a final bladder check, she burst out laughing when she saw me. By this time I was really getting into to the role of a Proton Warrior and was enjoying the attention. I then went to do my treatment and Shane also laughed full-heartedly when I walked into the treatment gantry wearing my warrior's costume. After treatment, Shane, Sara, Marci, and Marilyn, the technicians who delivered most of my treatment, came to the patient changing area where a number of my friends had gathered for my graduation. My good friend Henry, the stand up comic, stood beside me stealing some of my limelight with his well delivered jokes. Then it was time for my graduation and I led them all down the hall with Henry by my side. As we headed to the area where the gong was and where men gave their graduation speech, I saw the Latino cleaning lady with whom I occasionally spoke broken Spanish staring at me in disbelief. Waving to her I yelled out "Adios, me Amiga."

"Adios, mi amigo," the cleaning lady responded with a bright smile on her face.

I came to the double doors leading to the other hallway with the gong. Momentarily anxious and plagued again with self-doubt, I hesitated and then pushed the doors open and strode in with my friends trailing behind.

"He actually did it," I heard Pam, the wife of one of my friends gasped out as I walked in and they all laughed and applauded.

Facing me were 20 or so of my good friends, fellow proton warriors who faced the threat of prostate cancer with me and their lovely wives.

"Look at those bird legs," one of my male friends joked since he had heard me express concern over wearing a costume that exposed my spindly legs followed by laughter from the others.

Standing there in front of my friends, and celebrating the completion of my prostate cancer treatment, was a very heartwarming experience for me that is forever etched in my memory. Henry took the opportunity to give some good one-liners. I think he took advantage of the situation to steal some of my better jokes.

"Harold told me he is going to miss his morning routine of drinking coffee and then getting his balloon," Henry stated followed again by laughter.

I felt like I was high on drugs I was so elated. I don't remember exactly what I said but I thanked them all for coming, wished them all good luck, told them I would miss them, and then rang the gong.

After I rang the gong it was photo-taking time as I poised for my friends. I had given my camera to a friend who took the pictures in this section.

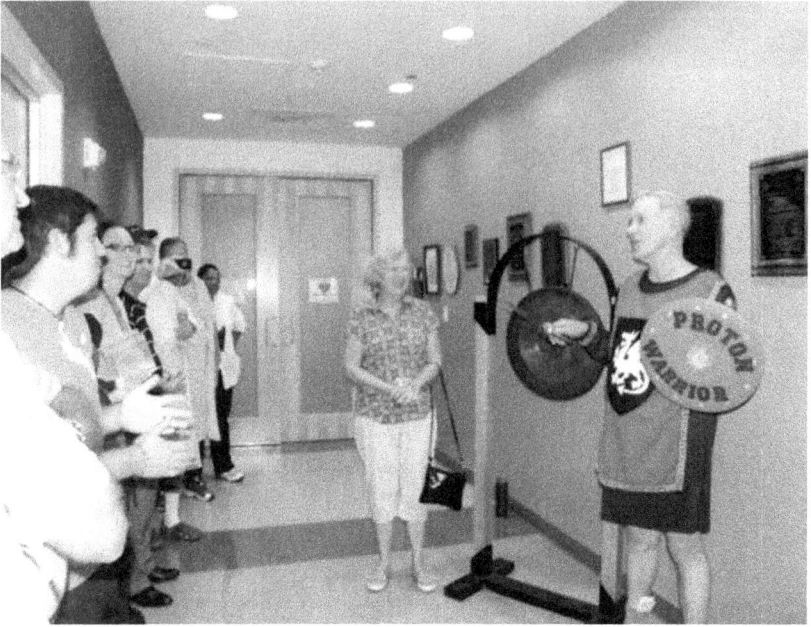

The original proton warrior graduates with his wife.

After eight weeks of daily treatment, I felt very close to the four technicians who administered my treatment and stood beside me below.

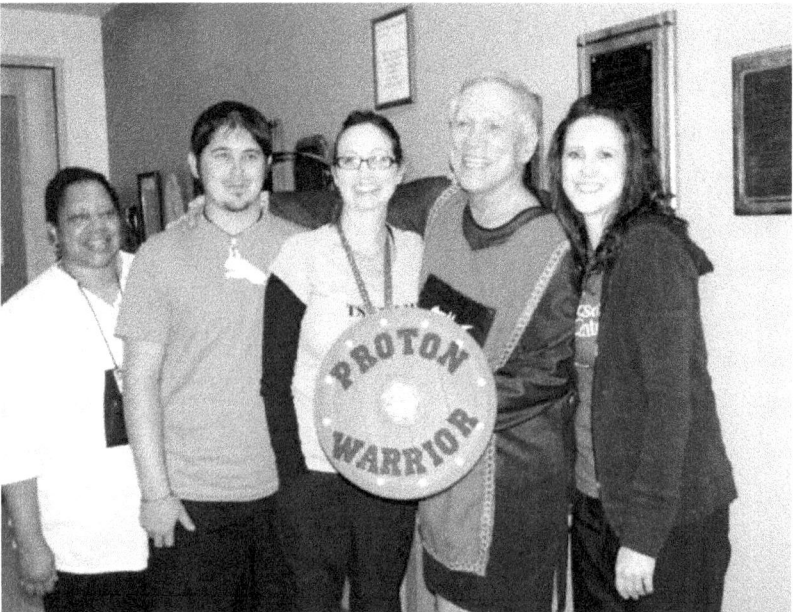

Marilyn, Shane, Marci, the original proton warrior, and Sara

My graduation ceremony was an enjoyable experience.

It was with a sense of sadness I returned to the changing room and dressed for the last time. I said my final goodbyes to my fellow proton warriors, shook hands all around, and, carrying my warrior costume, walked down the hall I had travelled along for the previous eight weeks. I then walked through the double doors where the gong was located, and into the large lobby waiting area at the base of the stairs. Several friends were still present and I said goodbye again to them and shook their hands. Linda and I then walked up the stairs, and stopping halfway up turned and took one last look down at the reception area below. A strange mixture of emotions swept over me. While I was certainly happy at having completed my treatment, the realization that I was leaving new friends with whom I had become close saddened me. Turning around Linda and I ascended the stairs and walked out of the Proton Therapy Center to our car parked in front.

Driving back to our home in Diamondhead, MS I kept thinking of the nice treatment staff and all of the friends we had made during my treatment. Linda felt the same way. She had also become friends with several of the wives of men going through treatment with me. One of her friends by the name of Pam also enjoyed shopping at thrift, consignment, and discount stores. I recalled the last dinner we had together and how Linda and Pam had dressed up with their "bling" consisting of costume jewelry they had bought from some of the discount stores in Houston.

It was time to return to our normal life.

Chapter Nine

The Incredible Effectiveness of

Proton Therapy

The best treatment with the least side effects.

Is Proton Therapy the New "Magic Bullet?"

In 1940 Edward G. Robinson starred in the classic film "Dr. Ehrlich's Magic Bullet," a movie based on the true story of Dr. Paul Ehrlich, a German physician credited with pioneering the use of dyes and other marking agents in the color staining and marking of certain cells and micro-organisms for diagnostic purposes. But Dr. Ehrlich is best known for his pioneering the use of certain chemicals via pill form or by injection to treat specific diseases, a process he referred to as "magic bullets." As Ehrlich searched for chemicals that could kill specific microorganisms responsible for certain infectious diseases such as syphilis and tuberculosis, he sought ways to do so without causing significant harm to the patient. There were plenty of chemicals and substances that could quickly kill bacteria but unfortunately they also either killed the patient or left the patient with painful side effects. Ehrlich eventually succeeded in developing one of the first effective chemotherapeutic agents that did not cause significant harm to the patient by injecting arsphenamine into the bloodstream of patients suffering with syphilis and he was able to cure them.

Ehrlich, like many other pioneers in the history of medicine, faced harsh criticism just as did Pasteur, Jonas Salk, among other medical pioneers. Proton therapy, like many other effective treatments in the history of medicine, is also being criticized unfairly by those who question its efficacy and claim its excessive costs make it impractical. History will prove them wrong.

Demonstrated Fewer Side Effects of Proton Therapy As Compared To Other Treatments

During the civil war physicians used the very effective procedure of preventing the death of men who had been severely wounded in the leg or arm by simply cutting the limb off. This approach worked and the men lived, plus it didn't take much time to do it. There only problem was the men were not happy with losing one or more of their limbs. The history of medicine is full of similar procedures that worked well in treating various diseases and injuries but had also very bad side effects. In the continuing advancement of medical science it is now possible to save a badly damaged limb by employing new and better procedures. In the treatment of prostate cancer almost all men receiving it will have their cancer controlled but many will do so at the price of producing bad side effects. And, just like new procedures became available to allow even severely damaged limbs to be saved, treatment is now available with results as good or better than all other treatments that allow prostate cancer to be cured WITHOUT the bad side effects common to the other procedures. That new treatment is proton therapy.

All credible treatments for prostate cancer produce equal and comparable results in curing the cancer. Most men with prostate cancer thus need to focus on treatments that produce the least side effects. There is clear evidence in terms of published research that proton therapy results in the least risk of serious side effects.

With over 90% of prostate cancer treatment done today is either surgery or conventional photon radiation and less than one percent is proton therapy, our discussion next will focus on side effects with these three treatments. The major side effects of prostate cancer treatments in general are (1) urinary and rectal incontinence, (2) erectile dysfunction, and (3) other problems. The risks of experiencing these side effects will be discussed relative to surgery, conventional photon radiation, and proton therapy.

Urinary Incontinence

A major problem in the treatment of prostate cancer field is the lack of specificity in defining urinary incontinence. According to Dr. Albert Vorstman, some urologists who treat prostate cancer surgically tend to use imprecise, non-scientific definitions such as "...incontinence may be defined as needing to wear more than two pads per day while impotence has been defined as being unable to engage in a sex act over a twelve month period." Dr. Vorstman added these imprecise definitions can be confusing for men seeking to understand the risk of incontinence associated with surgery and also serve the purpose of minimizing the side effects of surgery.[1]

Urinary incontinence is generally defined as the unintentional loss of urine due to the loss of voluntary control over the urinary sphincters resulting in the involuntary passage of urine. The bladder is a large balloon-like organ surrounded by muscle tissue and its purpose is to hold the urine as it is released from the kidneys. The urine leaves the bladder through a tube called the urethra. There are also muscles along the urethra and as they relax they allow the urine to flow through it.

The most common type of urinary incontinence after surgery is referred to as stress incontinence. This incontinence is caused by a sneeze or a cough, which triggers the release of urine. It occurs in as many as 60% of men who undergo surgery. Another type of incontinence is uncontrolled leakage. The wearing of an item such as a Depends pad commonly controls both of these types of urinary incontinence.

Urinary incontinence is the main side effect most men experience when they are treated for prostate cancer. Over 50% of men are directed to surgery and incontinence among these men can run as high as 60% or more. Men directed to conventional photon radiation such as Brachytherapy or IMRT also have a higher risk of urinary incontinence than men treated with proton therapy. When it does occur it is typified by the need for frequent urination along with episodes of excessive leaking.

Both surgery and conventional photon radiation disrupt the bladder and urethra, making it difficult for them to control urine. Conventional photon radiation exposes both the bladder and the rectum to more harmful radiation than experienced in proton therapy.

This radiation can decrease the bladder size and cause spasms that force the urine out. There are minimal risks of urinary incontinence associated with the treatment of prostate cancer using proton therapy. The ability to more precisely control and direct the proton beam to the tumor and its ability to then discharge its radiation energy results in little or no exposure to the bladder and other surrounding healthy tissue.

Urinary incontinence, if it does occur during or after proton radiation, generally happens in less than five percent of men and is usually temporary. During my eight weeks in treatment I did not encounter one patient who reported this problem.

Fecal Incontinence

While urinary incontinence is difficult to live with, fecal incontinence is an even more difficult problem. It is defined as the involuntary release of loose or solid stool and can be a devastating problem for men who experience it following treatment for prostate cancer. The problem again results from the higher amount of harmful radiation directed to the bladder and rectum during conventional photon radiation even using the more advanced IMRT procedures. While advancements have been made in the delivery of conventional photon radiation treatment of prostate cancer using IMRT, there is still the problem of the diffuse nature of this radiation and its resultant exposure to healthy tissue located near the prostate. The likelihood of fecal incontinence is closely related to the amount of harmful radiation received by the rectum. While the information available on the Internet is quite confusing as various sites each put their own spin on the degree of harm the rectum receives during conventional photon radiation or IMRT, there is unquestionable evidence that the amount of exposure is significantly greater than that received from proton therapy. An exhaustive review of the incidence of fecal incontinence following this type of radiation treatment for prostate cancer published in 2011 revealed the incidence can range from 1% to 58%.[2]. At this point any man seeking to avoid fecal incontinence needs to realize that regardless of how it is spun, the risk of experiencing this very serious problem is greater with conventional photon radiation. A similar risk of fecal incontinence was also found in a review study that reported an incidence of fecal leakage following surgical treatment of prostate cancer that ranged from 17% to 32%.[2,3].

The good news for men considering treatment for their prostate cancer is that there is a minimal risk of urinary or fecal incontinence with proton therapy.

Erectile Dysfunction - Impotence

Without question erectile dysfunction (ED, "male impotence") defined as sexual dysfunction characterized by the inability to develop or maintain an erection of the penis during sexual performance, is viewed by men as one of the most serious side effects following treatment for prostate cancer. This risk is especially high following surgery. This risk is so high that according to Dr. Vorstman, this term is also loosely used by some urologists who go to extremes such as defining a man as being sexually competent if he was able to maintain an erection once in six months or even once in 12 months.[1] Such misleading and confusing definitions serve the purpose of hiding the high risk of this problem occurring following surgery.

One of the difficulties in comparing the rate of erectile problems in surgery, IMRT, and proton therapy is the problem of age being a confounding variable. As men age there is a natural tendency for them to develop erectile problems. One study in men who had not received treatment for prostate cancer found that by age 40, 40% of men had erectile problems and that by age 70, 70% of men had such problems.[4] There are few studies on proton therapy and erectile dysfunction but the limited research that is available is encouraging.[5,6] One study of patients who were treated with proton therapy found that men under age 55 were sexually competent 18 months after treatment and had few side effects in general.[5]

According to Bob Marckini, who had his prostate cancer treated by proton therapy and who went on to form the patient fraternal group Brotherhood of the Balloon, sexual problems can occur in as many as seventy-five percent of prostate cancer patients treated with surgery. [7]In surgery, during the process of cutting out the prostate, it is very difficult not to damage the nerves associated with sexual pleasure. Very skilled surgeons using the procedure identified as "nerve sparing" may be able to protect this nerve from damage and the patient does not experience sexual problems. Because of the delicate nature of this procedure and the likelihood of sexual problems, the skill of the surgeon is the defining issue in a man selecting surgery. As pointed out earlier, not all surgeons have the skill level to ensure the nerves relating to sexual functioning are not damaged. There is also the issue of even a good surgeon having an off day. The net result is a high rate of sexual problems among men who have had surgery.

Erectile dysfunction is less of a problem for men treated with the advanced IMRT and proton therapy. The most significant indicator of ED occurring following the treatment of prostate cancer by either of these procedures is whether or not the man had good erectile functioning prior to treatment. The chances are good that men who had good erectile functioning prior to this treatment will continue to do so after treatment. Conventional photon radiation, other than the advanced IMRT, is likely to produce some sexual problems in about one-third of the patients. This results from the diffuse nature of conventional photon radiation harming healthy tissue including the nerves relating to sexual satisfaction. Advancements with IMRT have minimized the risk of erectile problems among men who select this treatment.

Some minor sexual problems may occur in patients who received either the advanced IMRT or proton therapy. The good news is that these problems tend to be less severe than experienced in patients having received surgery or other conventional photon radiation treatment. Most of these problems can be adequately treated with drugs such as Viagra and Cialais and that less than five percent develop serious sexual problems. But such drugs have a high risk of serious side effects including the risk of death. There are ways of minimizing ED following the treatment of prostate cancer with advanced IMRT or proton therapy. Furthermore, since men in general are at a higher risk of developing ED as they age, they too may be able to maintain their ability to engage in satisfactory sexual intercourse by using these same procedures.

Sexual problems are one of the most distressing side effects of prostate cancer. Because of the prevalence of this problem I decided to address it in more detail.

Keeping It Up – Erectile Fitness Training

While I was writing this book I was also fortunate to be working with my colleague Joel Block, Ph.D., who is a noted sex therapist and author of numerous successful books on sex. We had just finished the book *The New Sexually Assertive Woman – The Woman's Guide To Good Sex,*[8] a book written with our colleague Dr. Victoria Zdrok, intended to help woman derive more satisfaction in sex. I turned to my colleague for help in providing information on what men can do to maintain good erectile fitness after prostate cancer treatment. What developed is *Keeping It Up – Erectile Fitness Training,* presented in Appendix A. The simple fact to keep in mind is that the process of obtaining and maintaining an erection sufficient to engage in satisfactory sexual intercourse can be improved significantly for many men by engaging in regular sexual activity leading to orgasm at least two or three times a week. This process is referred to as Erectile Fitness Training (EFT) and facilitates the flow of blood carrying oxygen and nutrients to the blood vessels, tissues, and nerves associated with maintaining an erection and experiencing pleasure in sex. A more detailed explanation of EFT is provided in Appendix A.

Secondary Cancer from Radiation Treatment

Conventional photon radiation such as IMRT and Brachytherapy as well as proton therapy expose non-cancerous healthy tissue to radiation, which can damage the tissue. It is well known that radiation can cause cancer in cancer free tissue. It is thus important to keep in mind that proton therapy delivers only one-third the radiation delivered by conventional photon therapy. Proton therapy also delivers very little radiation as it enters the body by the use of medical physics and the unique characteristics of the proton beam as it deposits most of its radiation on the cancerous tumor and then immediately dissipates. By being able to deliver a very high dose of radiation to the cancer it is able to kill the cancer cells more effectively and at the same time delivering much less radiation to healthy tissue.

Radiation induced cancers can be reduced by as much as 39% when proton therapy is used instead of conventional photon radiation. The overall quality of life for proton therapy patients is greatly improved along with their having less risk of rectal, urethra problems, secondary cancers, and hip problems.[2]

Proton Therapy is a Magic Bullet

The verdict is in; proton therapy is a magic bullet in terms of treating certain types of cancer. It meets the age-old quest for ways of killing something that is harming us without causing great harm at the same time. Health care providers have long searched for a device or a procedure in which they could target the harmful entity without damaging surrounding tissue and organs. Since it is abundantly clear that proton therapy can be targeted to kill cancer effectively without damaging surrounding healthy tissue, it is thus a magic bullet. But still more is being done to enhance its effectiveness.

While erectile problems and incontinence can result in as many as 60% or more of men treated with IMRT or surgery, these problems seldom occur with proton therapy.

Research cited in this Chapter indicates the advantages of proton therapy over other treatments of prostate cancer.[10,11,12] Proton therapy delivers 35% less radiation to the bladder and 59% less radiation to the rectum in comparison with IMRT, which greatly minimizes the potential for side effects leading to incontinence and impotency. It takes twenty minutes of radiation exposure in IMRT while the proton therapy beam is delivered in eight seconds. While advancements have been made with the new versions of IMRT, this procedure still presents a risk to the bladder and rectum. The anterior wall of the rectum is so close to the prostate that it is very difficult to prevent spillover radiation from hitting it. Patients receiving IMRT subsequently have a greater risk of developing proctitis, a non-healing inflammation of the rectum from the burn of the conventional photon radiation. Symptoms may vary but can include rectal urgency, pain, bleeding, and incontinence.

Minimal Side Effects of Proton Therapy

Results from a University of Florida Proton Therapy Institute report show few side effects at 18 months following proton therapy treatment for prostate cancer among 98 men with low, intermediate, and high risk cancer. [10]

Summary of findings:

- 21 percent of patients experienced mild urinary side effects that were treated with prescription medication
- 3 percent experienced mild gastrointestinal side effects that were treated with prescription medication
- No patients experienced permanent incontinence
- No patients experienced significant rectal side effects
- 94 percent of those that did not receive androgen deprivation therapy were sexually active

- Only 2 patients were dissatisfied with their treatment decision

We are in the midst of an era of great strides being made in the treatment of prostate cancer and cancer care in general. In the forefront of these advancements are the remarkable successes being achieved by proton therapy. As more research on the effectiveness of proton radiation in treating certain cancers becomes available, it will emerge as the leading procedure for the treatment of pediatric malignancies, eye malignancies and disorders of the central nervous system, head and neck, urological, pulmonary, sarcoma, lymphoma, liver, lung, breast and prostate cancer. Gone will be the days when a diagnosis of breast cancer or a malignant brain tumor will amount to receiving a death sentence.

In the next twenty years significant advancements in the use of proton therapy, better ways of handling the movement of the target site during treatment, implementing more efficient and effective treatment planning, better use of image guided treatment, and treating additional types of malignancies will result in proton therapy emerging as one of the most widely used treatments for a number of different types of cancer.

The Importance of Quality of Life after Treatment

As an urologist with more than thirty-five years of experience in treating prostate cancer patients, Dr. Bert Vorstman states he has seen far too many men in despair after ending up with urinary incontinence and erectile problems stating "It is the fundamental act of cutting out from its location and association with the sphincter muscle fibers and nerves, whether conventionally or robotically, in high definition or with any other 'bells and whistles', that automatically gives rise to the common complications of impotence and incontinence."[1] He goes on to state "In fact, I believe these surgical treatment options represent a direct assault on manhood, and men choosing this radical surgical/robotic option for their prostate cancer are playing Russian roulette with the quality of their life." He further states "Hardly is it surprising then to hear some of these men afflicted with these horrible complications tell me that 'their' choice to have their prostate removed through radical surgery/robotics was 'the worst decision of my life' ".

Another vocal critic of how urologists treat prostate cancer is Dr. Bradley Hennenfelt, a physician and health economist. Writing in his book *The Big Lie in Surviving Prostate Cancer Without Surgery,*[13] Dr. Hennenfelt states "Urologists introduced radical prostate surgery without doing the necessary clinical studies. They went for money over science." An outspoken critic of the surgical treatment of prostate cancer, he goes on to state "The radical prostatectomy is a sacrifice, not a cure. Its rate of sexual dysfunction is a whooping 100 percent." In indicating how serious the side effect of this prostate cancer treatment can be, Dr. Hennenfelt describes the true case of one patient who was so devastated by these side effects that he went to the office of the urologist who performed the surgery and used a pistol to shoot him in the groin leaving him alive but impotent.

The Growing Attack on Proton Therapy

The billion-dollar prostate cancer industry is largely built on conventional photon radiation and surgery. As proton therapy becomes more popular and more people turn to it instead of other cancer treatments, those benefiting from those treatments face the threat of reduced income. Ominous signs are evident that unjustified attacks on proton therapy are growing. The first prong of these attacks is to discredit its effectiveness with the often-repeated criticism that "no controlled studies are available demonstrating its effectiveness over other treatments." The second attack is to argue it is too expensive, and the third prong is to claim it has a high risk of side effects. These attacks are well coordinated, appear to come from a variety of sources but may well originate from just a few sources, and are often repeated.

The "Lack of Controlled Studies" Argument: Even though this criticism also applies to the "other treatments" it is being relentlessly used to attack proton therapy. Repeating such a statement without acknowledging that it applies to the other prostate cancer treatments such as surgery and conventional photon radiation gives the erroneous impression that proton therapy is unique in that there is a lack of credible evidence that it is effective. It is well established that repeating a statement about a product, person or service, even one that is incorrect, a sufficient number of times can change how people perceive it. This practice is routinely used in politics to define opponents in a negative manner. Having a few statements that have been found to generate negative reactions when they are tested in focus groups repeatedly stated in the media or other settings is a common way of discrediting proton therapy. Those of us familiar with criticism of proton therapy know how often the statement "lack of controlled studies" is applied to proton therapy by advocates of competing treatments even when the treatments they advocate lack the same controlled studies.

The "It's Too Costly" Argument: The second prong of the attack is that proton therapy is too costly. Related to this argument are efforts to pressure Medicare and other funding for proton therapy to be cut. While proton therapy is more costly relative to other treatments, this difference in costs is diminishing as proton therapy machines are coming on the market that are smaller and less costly. As this trend continues, proton therapy will soon reach the point where its cost will be similar to that of conventional photon radiation treatment of prostate cancer. In addition, when the costs of dealing with the serious side effects resulting from less expensive prostate cancer treatments with risk of serious side effects are factored in, the difference in the overall cost may not be that significant.

The High risk of Side Effects Argument: It is common practice in business to directly attack the strongest advantage of a competing product or service. In politics, opposing politicians attack what voters most like about a politician. Such efforts can work by changing a positive into a negative. This approach can work well even when there is no factual support for it. Its purpose is to spread misinformation and inaccurate information about a competing product, service, or politician. It is designed to plant seeds of doubt in people's minds that previously held a positive view of what is now being unjustly attacked. Unfortunately, even when such false claims are disputed by facts, the damage is already done. This appears to be a new trend in the growing attack on proton therapy.

A Confusing Example of How Research Is Sometimes Presented

As I was finalizing this book, I saw reports of a study done by Dr. Ronald Chen, a radiation oncologist. I was fascinated by the way this research was described in the media. For example, an AP story on it was posted on USA Today online on 2-20-12[14] with the headline "Study Questions Proton Therapy for Prostate Cancer," a fairly alarming headline. The first sentence states "A warning to men considering a pricey new treatment for prostate cancer called proton therapy: Research suggests it might have more side effects than traditional radiation does," another alarming statement. This was followed by the second sentence "A study of Medicare records found that men treated with proton beams later had one-third more bowel problems, such as bleeding and blockages, than similar men given conventional radiation," apparently a report of the findings. Quickly following were statements unrelated to the research study but instead dealt with the cost of proton therapy. "It costs around $48,000 – at least twice as much as other prostate cancer treatments," was a typical statement. Then Dr. Ronald Chen is quoted as saying "There's no evidence that proton therapy is better for prostate cancer and the new results suggest it may cause more complications." These statements could give the impression that proton therapy may have a higher degree of side effects in general. I found myself wondering if readers would assume that this study not only found proton therapy patients reported a higher incidence of "bowel problems" but that it demonstrated a higher incidence of other side effects. A similar report was found online at the website HuffingtonPost.comOncologistTV.[15] The first sentence of this article states "A warning to men considering a pricey new treatment for prostate cancer called proton therapy: Research suggests it might have more side effects than traditional radiation does," another scary sentence that could lead people into believing it had a higher incidence of serious sides. Repeating the frequent criticisms against proton therapy the article added "Proton therapy is rapidly growing in use – Medicare covers it – even though no rigorous studies have tested whether it is as safe or effective as usual care." The article fails to mention that there is no such evidence supporting traditional radiation or surgery. A similar report in the Houston Chronicle, apparently based on the same press release, echoed similar statements.[16] This article quotes Dr. Chen as stating "Proton radiation is receiving a lot of attention as a new way to treat prostate cancer," and also quoting him as saying "It's the most expensive radiation technique today, but it is unclear if it actually improves patient outcomes."

I am not questioning the integrity of the reporters who wrote about Dr. Chen's research. I assume that the news reports cited were based on the press releases about it. I am also not criticizing Dr. Chen or his study. I am sure it will be a valuable addition to furthering the understanding of prostate cancer treatment. I also look forward to reading a full report when it is published in the Journal of the American Medical Association. It should be noted however, that this research has already been criticized for not following the standard classification of bowel problems. Thus, interpreting Dr. Chen's findings may be difficult. What I am pointing out here is how new research can sometimes be presented in press releases in biased ways. I don't know if this is what happened in the reporting of Dr. Chen's research but I am puzzled why so much negative emphasis was placed on the cost of proton therapy. The few media reports I've seen on Dr. Chen's study seemed more focused on making negative statements about proton therapy than on presenting detailed information on the results of his study. These reports appear to parrot the main criticisms against proton therapy. A few reports did briefly mention that IMRT had a higher rate of sexual problems associated with it. The reality is that the overwhelming majority of published research on proton therapy does not show it as having higher side effects than surgery or conventional photon radiation, a fact that seems to be challenged by the way the media reports were written.

No doubt there are some men who do have side effects from proton therapy but the published incidence of serious side effects of impotence, serious bowel problems, and incontinence is lower in this treatment compared with other treatments. It is probably not a valid comparison but what comes to my mind as I read the above news reports, all of which essentially make the same comments, is something like a newspaper headline screaming "Thousands Injured In Shipwreck." Such a statement can give the impression of a large number of seriously injured people. Such an impression could be further supported if the article with such a headline does not differentiate the degree of severity of those injured and instead just discusses the large number of people that are injured. This is how the reports of Dr. Chen's paper appear to me. The problem with the media reports on Dr. Chen's research (presumably based on the press releases he did or approved) is that there is, at least in ones I read, insufficient information to determine the meaning of his research findings. The AP Report of Dr. Chen's research discussed above[15] also quoted Dr. James Cox, an M.D. Anderson professor of radiation oncology, responding to its findings by stating "That's certainly contrary to everything I've seen and read in the literature of proton therapy." Dr. Cox added, "The rate of significant gastrointestinal side effects from proton therapy is usually very low." Dr. Cox also stated that Dr. Chen did not use the standard category for classifying bowel problems. Dr. Cox's last statement is crucial in understanding the point I am seeking to make.

If Dr. Chen's study does not differentiate the severity of the bowel problems and instead lumps them all together and labels them as "bowel problems," many if not most of these problems may be minor or even inconsequential. While Dr. Chen apparently differentiated side effects of early verses later, more advanced IMRT, he seems to have failed to do the same with proton therapy, grouping all patients who received this treatment together in one group. Since improvements have been made in delivering proton therapy in an improved manner to minimize side effects, one would expect that looking only at patients who went through this latter treatment would have a significantly lower incidence of bowel problems. The full publication of his research will hopefully provide a better understanding of type and severity of "bowel problems" reported in his research. The unfortunate point is that the press reports sent out to the media may have already given the general impression that proton therapy not only has a higher incidence of "bowel problems" without differentiating the severity of these problems as well as vague warnings of other serious side effects as well. A recent study in the Archives of Internal Medicine shows that when proton therapy is available near where men live it is their treatment of choice.[17] My concern is that as increasing numbers of men are turning to proton therapy to treat their prostate cancer, its success is threatening the vested interest of those in the other traditional ways of treating prostate cancer.

Chapter Ten

How Some Prostate Cancer Patients See Their Urologist

"The superior doctor prevents sickness; The mediocre doctor attends to impending sickness; The inferior doctor treats actual sickness."

Chinese Proverb

The Changing Physician-Patient Relationship

It was not that long ago when the main source of information we had for health problems was the physician treating us for that problem. We were dependent on him or her for this information and relied primarily on what he or she recommended in terms of treatment. With the advent of the Internet came many new sources of health information. A large and growing number of websites now exist where we can find detailed and accurate information on just about every health problem imaginable. In a matter of seconds we can search the web and find helpful information on specific health problems and the best ways of treating them. Numerous websites exist that provide excellent information to help us understand our health problems and facilitate decisions we make in how they are treated. Government sites such as the National Institutes of Health and non-profit sites such as the American Cancer Society are good sources for us to turn to in terms of seeking information about prostate cancer. While our physician still plays a major role in helping us to understand our health problems, we now have additional sources of

127

obtaining this information that better enable us to make an informed choice when we elect a treatment.

The net result of the availability of these additional ways of quickly obtaining accurate information about health problems is changing our relationship with physicians. Since we are no longer completely dependent upon them for information about our health problems, we have greater control over decisions we make in terms of how they are treated. By researching different treatment options we can become knowledgeable about the pros and cons of different treatments. Armed with this knowledge we are better able to make informed decisions when it comes to deciding how we want our health problem treated.

A problem can arise when a disparity exists between what we have learned on our own from going to reliable sources and what our treating physician recommends. In earlier times when we were dependent upon our physician for information on our health problems and how best to treat them, we invariably relied on his/her recommendations. We then generally followed whatever was recommended. It is a different story today. We are a better educated public and in many cases can acquire a sufficient amount of information to make our own treatment decisions regardless of what our physicians recommend. I did this when I selected proton therapy after my urologist recommended robotic surgery. Many other men are now taking charge of their health and are not blindly following whatever their urologist recommends in terms of how their prostate cancer will be treated.

Hopefully, this book will help you in taking charge of your health so that you make decisions that are in your best interest. In addition you will likely go to the Internet and search on your own for information on prostate cancer and the pros and cons of different treatments for it. Furthermore, you may have consulted with a medical oncologist or an Internist and acquired even more information. If you have taken any of these steps you will be better prepared to make the right decision in terms of what you want to do about your prostate cancer.

As a result of reading this book and perhaps other searches on the Internet, you will also have an awareness of the financial incentives that may sometimes be associated with various prostate cancer treatments. All of this information will empower you to take more control over your health. When we have such power we are better able to make decisions that are in our best interests.

What follows next is a discussion of a survey I did on proton therapy patients who were empowered by possessing such information and who took charge of their health by making decisions that were in their best interests.

Not Good News for Urologists

Early in my treatment I began to be become aware of the negative experiences many of the other patients had with the urologists who diagnosed their prostate cancer. Many of these patients reported that when they did not agree to accept surgery or conventional photon radiation their urologist or an associate provided, the urologists attitude changed to one less positive. As I later discovered, many of these patients were well educated and had invested a significant amount of time and effort researching prostate cancer and were knowledgeable about the various ways to treat it. This empowerment led them to conclude that proton therapy was an equally effective treatment that had the least risk of side effects. As a result of their knowledge, they experienced a disparity between what they knew and what their urologists were recommending. After hearing variants of this experience from a large number of patients, I decided to survey a sampling of patients going through treatment with me to obtain more detailed information. I also knew that since most of the patients had been recently diagnosed with prostate cancer, their memory of this experience would be fresh in their minds and easy to recall accurately. This chapter covers the results of this survey.

Description of Survey

Based on my discussions with fellow patients, I developed a 25-item survey questionnaire. I used the Internet survey service ConstantContact.com to distribute the survey and generate the results. I used e-mail addresses provided to me by one of the patients who had collected them by putting up a volunteer sign-up sheet in the patient changing area. Patients provided their names and email addresses on this sheet with the understanding that they were doing so to facilitate contact among one another. After I developed my survey, I then submitted the patient e-mail list to ConstantContact.com who then sent out my survey to the proton therapy patients. I explained that my survey was not sanctioned, approved, or supported in any way by MD Anderson and that it was something I was doing on my own. I further indicated that their participation was strictly voluntary. After they completed the survey their responses were sent back to ConstantContact.com who then compiled the results before sending them on to me. These results are discussed in this Chapter. Some comments added by patients are presented exactly as they were made with grammatical errors included.

High Response Rate

The first significant finding was the high response rate of 54% the survey generated. Constantcontact.com reports the normal response rate can be expected to range from 10% to 20%. A number of factors likely contributed to this high response rate with many of the patients knowing me personally likely being a major factor. Another important factor in this high response rate could well be the degree of dissatisfaction with the urologist who diagnosed their prostate cancer and their overall satisfaction with their experience in going through proton therapy.

The Findings

The number of the survey question or questions and some of the responses to them are provided next.

(1) What is your age?

Twelve percent of respondents were below age 55, a further 41% were below age 63, and adding everyone together under age 76 indicated 71% were below this age. A further twenty percent were between 70 and 75 years of age and the remaining 7.6% were aged 76 to 81.

(2) Years of education you completed:

The first significant finding from the survey was the large number of college graduates. Over 75% of the respondents were graduates of a four-year college program with 25% of them having obtained a postgraduate degree. According to Wikipedia, the 2005 percentage of college graduates from a four-year university in the United States is 27%.

(3) How many miles away is your home from the Proton Therapy Center?

Forty-three percent of patients reported living more that 501 miles from the Proton Therapy Center with 28.3% reporting they lived between 301 to 500 miles away, and 25% reporting they lived within 100 miles. One patient reported living outside of the United States.

(4,5) How much effort and time did you spend studying different treatment options?

Eighty-seven percent of respondents reported spending "Very much" or "Much" time studying different treatment options for prostate cancer. In terms of the number of hours spent studying different treatments, 4 reported less than 10 hours, 9 reported 11 to 21 hours, with 26 reported spending 22 to 43 hours or more studying different treatment options. To quantify the time, over 55% reported spending in excess of 33 hours studying different treatments. These findings suggest that these patients invested a great deal of time and effort learning about different prostate cancer treatments.

(6) How long ago were you first diagnosed with prostate cancer?

Eighty-seven percent of the respondents reported having been diagnosed with prostate cancer within the last year and 61.4% reported that they were diagnosed within the preceding seven months.

(7) This question contained an error and is not reported, as it was confusing to many patients.

(8) What was the specialty of the physician who first diagnosed your prostate cancer?

Thirty-eight of the 39 respondents identified the physician who diagnosed their prostate cancer and recommended treatment as an urologist.

(9) What treatment did the physician who first diagnosed your prostate cancer recommend? Please check all that apply.

Sixty-six percent of the patients reported that their urologist recommended surgery with another 35.8% reporting conventional photon radiation was recommended and 10.2 % reporting that Brachytherapy was recommended. Almost 18% reported that watchful waiting was recommended. None of the patients reported that their urologist recommended proton therapy. It should be noted that some urologists recommended more than one treatment so the percentages on this question do not add up to 100%.

(10) Do you personally know someone who had surgery for prostate cancer and is now experiencing urinary incontinence?

Almost 58% (57.8) of the patients reported that they personally knew someone who had surgery for their prostate cancer and are now experiencing urinary incontinence.

(11) Did the physician who first diagnosed your prostate cancer express any opinion about proton therapy?

Thirty percent of the respondents reported that their urologist expressed negative views toward proton therapy with an additional 43% reporting that their urologist did not express any opinion about proton therapy.

Some comments to this question:

"Told me to never come back to him if I had proton therapy and that he knew 2 people who went to California for proton therapy and they 'burned his inside'…"

"Urologist said the proton beam might hit areas it was not supposed to hit."

"he called it 'the new glitzy ball.' Said no evidence that it worked. Said that it didn't work for any of his patients in his support group. Wife said, 'of course, if it worked they wouldn't be in the group.' Also said if he had cancer he'd go to Anderson, but then wouldn't refer us for anything but his surgery or surgery by a friend of his."

(12) Do you believe the physician who diagnosed your prostate cancer and recommended treatment other than proton therapy was influenced by factors other than those that were in your best interest?

A surprising 46.1% of the patient responded yes to this question. Another 33% responded that they were not sure. Only 17.9% responded no.

Some comments to this question:

"Small town, believe Urologist and local Radiation Oncologist were a 'team' and probably owned the equipment together."

"He did not know me well. He was very kind and offered great support and information regarding the disease but not the treatment options."

"The practice he worked in was owned by the surgeon he sent me to."

"I had a feeling that she knew about Proton Therapy and didn't want to recommend it."

"Physicians who recommend treatment which they offer....are like superior athletes, meaning that they must believe that they are the best. Unfortunately this means that they may not recognize that other treatments may be better."

"He was new in town and the only urologist in town. He had a monthly surgery quota to meet at the hospital to retain his ability to do surgery. It is the only hospital in the region. I think that motivated him to press for surgery."

"His office was affiliated with a traditional radiation center."

(13) Do you know of someone who went through surgery for his prostate cancer and is now sexually impotent?

Forty-three percent (43.5%) of them reported that they knew of someone who went through prostate cancer surgery who is now sexually impotent. Almost sixty percent (53.8%) responded no.

Some comments to this question:

"Did not ask, but many had other issues – rectal bleeding and other issues."

"The urologist did say it was a 100% of permanent impotence then implied I was 60 so really not a big thing anyway."

"This individual had robotic surgery a few months ago and is now suffering from both incontinence and impotence – may not be permanent. He doesn't know."

(14) Have you read or heard secondhand reports about other men who had surgery for their prostate cancer and experienced sexual problems following the surgery?

Eighty-two percent reported that they had heard about men who had sexual problems following prostate cancer surgery.

(15) How important to you was it to select a treatment that cured your prostate cancer with the least side effects?

In terms of the importance they place on finding a treatment that cured their prostate cancer with the least side effects, 38 of the

39 respondent reported it was "Very important" with the 39th patient reporting it was "Important."

(16) Do you feel that the physician who first recommended treatment described the side effects associated with that treatment in a complete and accurate manner?

Forty-one percent of respondents reported that they believed the urologist who diagnosed their prostate cancer and then recommended treatment did not describe the side effects of the treatment they recommended in a complete and accurate manner.

(17) Did the physician who diagnosed your prostate cancer tell you that proton therapy has the same side effects commonly associated with traditional photon radiation therapy?

Almost 72% (71.7%) responded no. Twenty-three percent of them reported that they were told that proton therapy treatment for prostate cancer had the same side effects commonly associated with conventional photon therapy.

(18) If the physician who diagnosed your prostate cancer recommended traditional radiation (non-proton) and/or surgery, do you believe he/she had a conflict of interest if he/she stood to experience financial gain if you selected the treatment he/she recommended?

Fifty-percent of respondents reported they believed the urologist who diagnosed their prostate cancer and then recommended a treatment had a conflict of interest if they stood to experience financial gain. A further 31% reported that they were not sure if there was a conflict of interest, and only 15.7% reported that they did not believe it represented a conflict of interest.

(19) Did the attitude of the physician who first diagnosed your prostate cancer change after you indicated you were NOT going to follow his/her treatment recommendations?

Over one out of four respondents (26.3%) reported that their urologist seemed displeased when they did not agree to follow their treatment recommendations. Thirty nine percent (39.4%) reported no change in his/her attitude.

Some comments to this question:

"It became a challenge to get my urologist office to send med records and biopsy to MD Anderson. Several request had to be made. The doctor never made any comments."

"Displeased is putting it lightly. He only offered to refer us to a "friend in Seattle" after I refused his surgery."

"Never saw the guy again after the initial diagnosis."

"DR. SENT WORD BY THE NURSE THAT I DIDN'T NEED TO COME BACK THERE AGAIN, IF I WAS GOING TO MDA"

(20) If the physician who first diagnosed your prostate cancer seemed displeased when you did not accept his/her treatment recommendations do you feel part of this displeasure was related in anyway to lost income he/she would have generated from the recommended treatment?

Only 22% of the patients reported that they believed that the treatment recommendation was primarily made on what the physician thought was best for them. Sixteen percent (16.6%) believe that lost income was a major factor in their urologist's displeasure and an additional 19.4% believed it was a minor factor in their displeasure. Twenty-five percent reported they did not know.

(21) Has your experience with the physician who first diagnosed your prostate cancer changed the way you now view physicians?

In terms of whether or not their experience with the urologist who first diagnosed their prostate cancer changed how they now view physicians, 58.9% reported no change. Thirty-three percent (33%) reported that it has resulted in a more negative view.

Some comments to this question:

"I expect a specialist, like the urologist, to be informed but not necessarily expert in all treatments related to his area of specialty. I believed before this that a patient should not have blind trust. My experience proves that patients need to do their own research to make informed decisions on treatments best for them."

"It was approx 6 weeks after my biopsy before I was told I had prostate cancer."

"I used to think you 'went to the doctor to get better'. I used to believe that doctors were fully knowledgeable in their field(s) of study, and would KNOW what was best for the patient. I now mistrust doctors. I now take a doctor's feedback as 'opinion' only, and feel the need to use that opinion as a focal point to begin my own research. This is not only for prostate cancer, but for all health issues."

(22) Has your experience with the physician who first diagnosed your prostate cancer changed your level of trust in physicians?

Thirty-four percent of them reported that their experience with the urologist who first diagnosed their prostate cancer has resulted in their having less trust toward physicians.

Some comments to this question:

"I was already suspicious of some of them, but had only seen this Urologist twice"

"I'm not a very trusting person. Reality is for most people that outside a small circle of people, no one really knows what happens to you anyhow."

"What I believe is a physician has an obligation to keep informed on new treatments relative to their specialty and help their patient with research and to make an informed decision."

"I am a firm believer in second or ever third opinions. Especially when it comes to life threatening illnesses."

"No reason to feel differently."

"my continuing experience with physicians is that they are human, have a lot or other patients, and have limited experience. One must always look out for yourself"

(23) Do you believe physicians have an ethical responsibility to inform their patients when they have a financial investment in the assessment or treatment services they are recommending?

Ninety-two percent of respondents reported they believe physicians have an ethical responsibility to inform patients when they have a financial investment in the assessment and/or treatment services they are recommending.

Some comments to this question

"An honest assessment is all I expect. If a physician tells me his recommendation is based on what he or she does, I fine with that. I would like to hear about other options, but wouldn't expect a lot of detail."

"Provided they are aware and believe that equal or superior treatments (with less side effects) are available elsewhere. Ignorance, intentional or otherwise, should not be an option for a professional"

"Physicians are in the business of improving patients' health. That is also how they make a living. We all already know that a physician's recommendation to treat the patient him/herself will result in income. It is unnecessary to further inform patients of this fact."

"But come on, do you really think that they are going to take money out of there pockets? Hell no"

Absolutely"

"Or research interest"

"But like politicians. It will never happen. I am not a cynic, just a realist"

(24) Do you believe most physicians tell their patients when they have a financial investment in assessment and/or treatment services they recommend?

Close to Ninety percent (89.7) of the respondents reported that they don't believe most physicians inform their patients when they have a financial investment in assessment or treatment procedures they are recommending.

Some comments to this question:

"Let's not get silly. Making money in large obscene sums is the scared cow in this country. People's welfare is secondary no matter what the business."

"Particularly urologists"

"Don't know"

"I believe the entire medical profession is money driven. Physicians do not spend enough time with patients to get to know their bodies and determine the root cause of many ailments. They over prescribe medication and most patients are foolish enough to believe chemicals can heal all of their ailments. Most patients are too lazy to do what is necessary to achieve optimum health. Think pills will fix every thing."

"It would be expected however. They do not work for nothing."

"Good reputable Physicians would always make that disclosure. Mine did it by saying He would do the Surgery ie he profits, and said the IMRT he would recommend was owned by his group. Did not out and out say he would profit, but between the lines you should know."

(25) Do you believe physicians should be required to inform their patients when they have a financial investment in assessment or treatment procedures they are recommending?

Ninety-two percent of the respondents reported that they believed that physicians should be required to inform their patients when they have a financial investment in assessment or treatment services they are recommending.

Discussion – Why Some Prostate Cancer Patients Don't Trust Their Urologist

One of the significant findings of this survey was the degree of distrust the patients felt toward the urologist who diagnosed their prostate cancer. These patients reported that even though surgery and/or conventional radiation were recommended by their urologists, they selected proton therapy. Forty six-percent believed their urologist was influenced by factors other than those that were in their best interests in recommending treatment for their prostate cancer. Forty-one percent believed their urologist did not describe the side effects of the treatment they recommended in a complete and accurate manner. Their experience with their urologist left 33% with a more negative view of physicians with 34% reporting their experience resulted in their having less trust toward physicians. Based on these circumstances one can't help but understand why so many distrusted their urologist.

This survey is likely the first assessment of patients who did not accept the treatment recommendations of the urologist who diagnosed their prostate cancer. This survey also revealed an educated and informed group of patients with 75% having a four year college degree or higher as well as having spent "very much" or "much" time researching different prostate cancer treatments. Every one of these patients reported that finding a treatment with the least side effects was the most important factor. Based on their own research they selected proton therapy as opposed to the treatment recommended by their urologist. These survey results also indicate a strong belief that physicians should be required to inform patients when they have a financial investment in assessment or treatment services they recommend. These findings suggest that when patients carefully research and study various treatments of prostate cancer, most tend to select ones that are minimally invasive such as proton therapy.

Conclusion

Based on the reports of patients that their urologist was either not aware of proton therapy or elected not to tell them it was an option for them to consider, the question arises if this failure was based on a bias against it or ignorance on the part of the physician. Either reason does not reflect well on urologists as the patients were able to become quite knowledgeable about the benefits of proton therapy in a relatively short period of time. Their self-education led to self-empowerment, which led to their selecting proton therapy. They were aware of the high risks of side effects with the treatments recommended and made the decision to go with proton therapy because it had the least risk of side effects. The distrust of physicians patients reported in this survey is understandable based on the discrepancy between what they have learned from independent and objective sources about the various treatments of prostate cancer and the treatment recommended by the urologist who diagnosed their prostate cancer.

Chapter Eleven

Surviving the Perils of the Prostate Cancer Industry

There can be a difference between how well a treatment works for you and how well it works for your doctor.

The New Prostate Cancer Marketplace

"In my experience, doctors play down punishing side effects like incontinence, impotence and shrinking of the penis. Those are just words when you hear them, but beyond language when you go through them."[1]

Dana Jennings, The New York Times Reporter in reference to his prostate cancer surgery

The new prostate cancer marketplace is a perilous setting. Dominated by the Prostate Cancer Industry, it is fraught with pitfalls and dangers to which many men fall victim. Safe havens do exist, as there are plenty of urologists and treatment facilities that have the best interests of their patients in mind. I was fortunate in having found both. Men must exercise caution upon entering this marketplace.

Those of us with prostate cancer soon discover that we are highly sought after customers as urologists and treatment facilities compete with each other to provide their own treatment to us. Major marketing efforts are directed to us with the market leaders being providers of surgery and IMRT. To survive in this marketplace, we must carefully shop for the best prostate cancer treatment with the least side effects.

This is our period of greatest vulnerability and regrettably is also the time when we are subjected to the greatest pressure to select treatments that may not be in our best interests.

The Controversial Issue of Physician Self-Referral

The key period of vulnerability for men being steered into prostate cancer treatments with a high risk of side effects is when they are still under the care of the urologist who diagnosed their cancer. These newly diagnosed men turn to this urologist with trust and respect assuming they will receive objective information based on their needs and not the needs of the urologists. The danger comes from the growing trend among urologists to buy into expensive robotic surgery and/or IMRT devices or facilities and refer patients they just diagnosed to themselves or an associate for treatment using these devices. Since the majority of prostate cancer treatment is provided directly or indirectly by urologists, the financial implications of self-referral are obvious. Medical oncologist Dr, Mark Scholz states that through years of experience physicians have a subtle yet effective way of influencing patients into selecting the treatment they recommend. When it is prostate cancer and the physician is an urologist, surgery is what they usually recommend. Dr. Scholz goes on to state that this critical moment of decision usually passes without patients adequately considering the different treatments or their side effects. According to Scholz, "A decision to do surgery is often made without the patient realizing how biased his surgeon-advisor is in favor of operating. Men don't realize that through experience and practice, doctors develop a persuasive, soft sell approach; everything about their demeanor and body language conveys the message that surgery is the best treatment. Most men never understand these dynamics until it's too late."[2]

Men with newly diagnosed prostate cancer are extremely vulnerable and many place their complete trust in the hands of the urologist who diagnosed them. Urologist Dr. Bert Vorstman is blunt in describing the influence urologists have on men shortly after they have diagnosed their prostate cancer when he states "Furthermore, many physicians in this medical business have become quite adept at persuading and insincerely coddling patients and purposefully fostering concern in order to manipulate the patient to follow a treatment path of no or marginal benefit to himself, but of every benefit to the doctor."[3]

Since most urologists are trained as surgeons their tendency to recommend surgery is understandable. Improvements have also been made in IMRT so their investment in it is also understandable. The risk of side effects from these two treatments can be so severe many men who experience them report they would have preferred taking their chances with untreated cancer. It is truly unfortunate that so little time and effort is spent on fully educating and informing men about the risk of serious side effects these treatments have along with their not being sufficiently informed about other treatments that have minimal risk of serious side effects.

Not only is criticism coming from health care professionals, the popular media is raising concerns about the financial implications of physician self-referral. The New York Times reporter Gina Kolata wrote an interesting article titled "Results unproven, robotic surgery wins converts" in the 2-14-10 issue. Discussing the amount of money made in the robotic surgical treatment of prostate cancer, Kolata quotes a physician at a leading medical center as saying "With the stream of prostate cancer patients that come through.... this is a big, big business." Kolata quotes another physician associated with a leading medical center as saying "...once a hospital invests in a robot - $1.39 million for the machine and $14,000 a year for the service contract...it has an incentive to use it. Doctors and patients become passionate advocates, assuming that newer means better."[4]

With increasing numbers of urologists entering into joint ownership arrangements for treating prostate cancer with IMRT, there also appears to be a clear financial incentive to refer to this treatment. The Washington Post reporter Rob Stein, writing in the 2-28-11 article discussing IMRT "Doctor-owned centers spark criticism, scrutiny," stated "Critics charge that they are a disturbing development in an alarming trend: doctors in many specialties referring patients to facilities in which they have a financial interest, possibly leading to unneeded and sometimes dangerous procedures and adding to the nation's bloated medical bill." Stein goes on to describe concerns from various regulatory agencies over this trend. He quotes one health care executive as stating "I think it is one of the biggest scandals in America today" adding "Do you want your dad going to somebody who has a very incentivized reason to give him one particular treatment that is not necessarily in his best interest?"[5]

Two reporters with The Washington Post, John Carreyrou and Maurice Tamman wrote an interesting 12-7-10 article titled "A device to kill cancer and lift revenue." Pointing out the loophole inserted into legislation intended to protect the public from abuses related to physician self-referral, they state "Taking advantage of an exemption in a federal law governing patient referrals, groups of urologists across the country have teamed up with radiation oncologists to capture the lucrative reimbursements IMRT commands from Medicare." They further state "Under these arrangements, the urologists buy radiation equipment and hire radiation oncologists to administer it. They then refer their patients to their in-house staff for treatment. The bulk of Medicare's reimbursements go to the urologists as owners of the equipment." They further cite James Mohler, a urologist at Roswell Park Cancer Institute in Buffalo, N.Y., who chairs a physicians' committee that sets national treatment guidelines for prostate cancer, as stating "Overtreatment with IMRT is a fact." They further quote Dr. Mohler as citing a 2006 study in the Journal of the National Cancer Institute that found that 45% of American men with prostate cancer who received external radiation were being over treated. They state further: "A Journal analysis of Medicare claims suggests that IMRT usage is significantly higher in the five states where most of the urology groups that own radiation equipment are located. These states—New York, Florida, Pennsylvania, New Jersey and Texas—are home to 22 of the 37 self-referral groups identified by the Journal. The average IMRT usage for recently diagnosed prostate-cancer patients was 42% in those states in 2008. By contrast, the national average was about a third." These reporters go on to cite statistics showing a marked increase in billing to Medicare in localities after urology groups begin offering IMRT. They go on to state scrutiny of urology groups involvement with IMRT has been spurred on by the "American Society for Radiation Oncology, or ASTRO, which has denounced urologists' practice of referring patients for treatment in facilities they own as unethical."[6]

The New York Times reporter Stephanie Saul writing in an article titled "Profit and questions on prostate cancer therapy" summed up the issue of urologist treatment decisions being influenced by financial factors. She cited concern among other physicians who worry that IMRT is but another example how financial incentives can influence treatment decisions and quotes Dr. Brian Moran, a radiation oncologist as stating "It's all money driven, and it's a shame medicine has come down to this." She goes on to also quote Dr. Eli Glatstein, a Professor of Radiation Oncology at the University of Pennsylvania expressing his concern that some urologists who steer patients to treatment could greatly profit from as stating, "It's not illegal to do this," and then adding "That doesn't make it right." Saul goes on to cite statistics that IMRT carries a risk of impotence stating "A recent study at Memorial Sloan-Kettering Cancer Center, which has conducted much of the early research on the therapy, found that eight years after treatment, 49 percent of men who were potent before treatment developed erectile problems."[7]

Critics of how physician self-referral is being abused don't have a problem with how much money urologists make. They know that physicians work hard to obtain their medical education and have the right to earn money, even a great deal of it. The important issue to those of us who develop prostate cancer is that it be successfully treated without leaving us with serious side effects. There is also concern over unnecessary treatment resulting in health care costs to soar and Medicare expenditures to explode.

The trend of urologists buying into expensive medical devices and then engaging in self-referral will continue and likely expand. It is part of the changing medical marketplace and we will have to adjust to it. Urologists are now among the top five highest paid medical specialties with their average income for 2010 reported as $305,000 by Medscape from WebMD.com. This same report indicated that 14% of urologists earned in excess of $500,000 in 2011.[8]

Major efforts are underway from manufacturers of robotic surgery and IMRT devices encouraging urologists to purchase or otherwise become involved financially with treatment devices they manufacture. These devices are then aggressively marketed as the best treatment available. Urologist Dr. Albert Vorstman criticizes surgery including robotic surgery by stating "With the endorsement from some surgeons, the runaway juggernaut of surgical technology business and its support cast of financially motivated lobbyists have managed to "approve" for mainstream use, through very clever marketing, a very profitable but non-FDA scrutinized treatment option."[3]

In a 7-16-10 Washington Post article titled "Robotic surgery extends its reach in health care, hospital marketing" reporter Christine Torres describes the large investments being made by hospitals in purchasing robotic surgery devices. She quotes several physicians, one of whom states that competition is on "the level of billboards, advertisements, websites and more" and others physicians who point out the close relationship many hospitals have with manufactures of the robotic devices."[2]

Dr. Vorstman is also critical of the misleading marketing involved with robotic surgery by stating "...the complications and negative effects on quality of life by the radical surgical/robotic option appear to be intentionally minimized and clouded by manufacturer marketing spin."[3]

To those who may brush these concerns aside by stating that physicians have a right to earn a living, making money is not the issue. The issue is instead that of disclosure. Some physicians do not appear to be disclosing to their patients when they have a financial investment in services they are recommending. The significance of this issue may become more apparent if, for example, we think about how we would feel to discover that a financial advisor we were paying to recommend ways for us to earn the greatest return on our money with the least amount of risk stood to gain financially when we selected the investment he/she was recommending over other investments in which he did not stand to gain financially. How would we feel if we also discovered that the investments he did not recommend produced equally good returns with significantly less risks?

A pervasive factor evident in my survey discussed in Chapter Ten is the negative perception patients had toward their urologists who sought to refer them to treatment he/she provided. Physician self-referral is likely the major factor in the high degree of negativity the patients reported toward their urologists on the survey discussed in Chapter Ten. The specific cause of this negativity may well be the issue of physicians not disclosing their potential financial gain when they recommend specific treatment. About ninety percent (89.7%) of the patients reported they don't believe most physicians tell their patients when they have such a financial investment in the treatment they recommend. There does seem to be an awareness in organized medicine of the importance of physicians disclosing information about their financial investment in treatment services they recommend, as evidenced by the June 2009 AMA policy statement on ethics that physicians must "Disclose their financial interest in the facility, product, or equipment to patients; inform them of available alternatives for referral; and assure them that their ongoing care is not conditioned on accepting the recommended referral" (Issued June 2009 based on the AMA report " Physician Self-Referral CEJA 1-I-08," adopted November 2008).[10]

If physicians simply told their patients when they had a financial investment in services they were recommending, there would be less of a problem. There is a problem because many physicians don't make this disclosure and laws and regulatory efforts to force them to do so have been so weakened by the prostate cancer industry lobbyists as to nullify their basic intent. When questions are raised about the potential for abuse with physician self-referral, it is not unusual for one of the responses to be "It is not illegal to do so." So that leaves us with the responsibility of acquiring our own knowledge base and, to the extent possible, making our decisions based on what we know.

The Financial Implications of the Use of the PSA Test

On 10-7-11 a significant seismic event shook the prostate cancer industry when a draft report released by the Health and Human Services Department's Preventive Services Task Force[11] stated that routine use of the PSA for prostate-cancer screening does not save sufficient lives to justify exposing men to risks of side effects such as death, incontinence and impotence related to treatment. Since over 85% of men receive surgery and/or conventional photon radiation in the form of IMRT or Brachytherapy, these risks must assume to be related to these treatments. This task force recommended not using the PSA test unless men have symptoms that are "highly suspicious for prostate cancer."

One possible explanation for the increased profits from treating prostate cancer is that the PSA does, as proponents of its reduced use argue, lead many more into treatment than before its widespread use. While it has undoubtedly saved the lives of some men by their having treatment early who could have died from prostate cancer, it is the single most important factor contributing to increased rate of treatment and resultant risk of serious side effects. Opponents of the routine use of the PSA in screening healthy men argue that if this practice is stopped much of the overtreatment will stop.

The use of the PSA test is mainly criticized because of the large number of men who suffer side effects from prostate cancer treatment initiated by its use. Its use in screening healthy men can lead to more men receiving treatment that do not need it. The financial incentives inherent in urologists' self-referring patients they diagnose with prostate cancer to treatment they or an associate provide are a confounding issue in this ongoing debate. Those who benefit financially from the increased numbers of men receiving treatment resulting from the routine use of the PSA can have difficulty explaining what to some may be seen as an apparent conflict of interest from related financial incentives that apply directly to them if this current policy continues.

In 2002, two physicians, Dr. Gavin Yamey, and Dr. Michael Wilkes, wrote an opinion piece in the 1-18-02 Open Forum Section of the San Francisco Chronicle titled "Prostate cancer screening – is it worth the pain?"[12] These two physicians pointed out the absence of evidence supporting the routine use of the PSA in healthy men. Their article generated significant backlash. In a subsequent article available on the Internet these two physicians described how they were attacked for expressing their professional opinions on the use the PSA. The most aggressive response for such routine screening use has come from those that benefit financially from its use and their proxies. Proxies included a non-profit patient advocacy group who received significant funding from those benefitting from the continued of the PSA for routine screening in healthy men. In explaining why their opinion generated so much opposition, these authors made the following point: "More importantly, we dared to tread on the toes of the powerful pro-screening lobby. In encouraging all healthy men to take the PSA test, this lobby has a major conflict of interest since they receive funds from manufacturers of prostate cancer treatments or have ties with them."[13]

A European study that looked at the relative value of screening use of the PSA found it had little benefit. The researchers determined that 48 men who are not at risk of dying from prostate cancer would have to be treated for screening to prevent one death from the disease over nine years. The bottom line is that 48 men would risk the side effects of treatment to save one life.[14]

A study by H. Gilbert West, MD and Peter Albertsen, MD published online in the August 31 issue of the *Journal of the National Cancer Institute* reported that 1.3 million men were diagnosed with prostate cancer that wouldn't have been discovered without the PSA initiative, and more than 1 million of these men were treated between 1986 and 2005. Factoring in the rate of death from prostate cancer, the study reported that for every one man who avoids a death, more than 20 men and as many as 50 had to be over diagnosed and treated needlessly. Over-treatment would not be a problem were it not for the very adverse side effects associated with much of it. The study concluded, "Maybe one-third will have treatment problems such as impotence or incontinence."[15]

As a result of these complications, the man who developed the test, Dr. Richard J. Ablin, has called its widespread use a "public health disaster."[16] In this Op Ed article Ablin goes on to state "The medical community must confront reality and stop the inappropriate use of P.S.A. screening. Doing so would save billions of dollars and rescue millions of men from unnecessary, debilitating treatments."

Dr. Otis Brawley, the Chief Medical and Scientific Officer for the American Cancer Society has come out in support of the Health and Human Services Department's Preventive Services Task Force recommendations in a statement on CNN.com. Dr. Brawley goes on to state: "With evangelical fervor, true believers conducted mass screening in shopping malls, at state fairs and in supermarket parking lots. Medical practices, hospitals, drug and medical device companies, politicians and even manufacturers of adult diapers have sponsored screening. Most of these sponsors wanted to do a public service, but many profited from it. Some may also have been blinded by that profit."[17]

In a recent editorial Dr. Ablin states the two-fold increase in the over-diagnosis and over-treatment of more than a million men is directly related to the improper use of the PSA test he developed. He states that the "science" of the PSA test was extrapolated beyond its capabilities and points out it is not cancer specific in that it does not identify cancer. He states it is, instead prostate specific and its use in identifying prostate cancer is "slightly better than the flip of a coin." He also questions the value of biopsies triggered by the use of the PSA test citing research showing that "45% to 80% of men screened between ages 50 and 75 posses latent (histologic) asymptomatic cancer adding that in such biopsies cancer may well be found. He clarifies his view by stating in the average population of healthy men over half will posses latent, non-life threatening prostate cancer that does not need to be treated. Ablin further argues that another serious weakness of the PSA test is its inability to distinguish between prostate cancer that could kill verses prostate cancer that which is unlikely to harm us. In terms of the resultant "score" from the PSA test Ablin states there "is no single or absolute level of PSA definitive for prostate cancer." Ablin then asks "What if anything does it tell us relative to the purpose of screening for prostate cancer?" [18]

"Astroturfing" - Phony Patient Advocacy and Support Groups Funded By the Medical Industrial Complex

* * * * *

Bill, a retired factory worker, sat in his comfortable overstuffed recliner enjoying the morning news. During a commercial break an advertisement appeared that sort of looked like a public service announcement. It began with a video of an average appearing middle aged man surrounded by his children and grandchildren. It was a moving, loving scene that touched Bill. A calm voice began as the family scene continued "Joe has cancer and it may kill him unless he receives treatment. Effective treatment is available but congress is blocking Joe from receiving it. Call your Senators and Congressman and tell them you want them to support the Senate Bill to allow Joe to receive the help he needs." As images of Joe and his family slowly fade a voice states "Call now and voice your support for Joe. His family needs him." A different voice then states "This announcement was funded by Patients for Better Cancer Treatment, a non-profit organization focused on improving cancer treatment." Moved by what he saw Bill picks up the phone and calls his Senators and Congressman and tells them to support the bill to help Joe live.

* * * * *

The above is not a true story. It is a fictitious example of how an Astroturf organization set up by a segment of the medical-industrial complex achieves its goals. I made up the group "Patients for Better Cancer treatment" but because there are so many Astroturf groups being set up masquerading as non-profit grass root patient organizations any similarity to an existing group is strictly by chance. In the example above, Congress was considering reforms to Medicare including efforts to limit unnecessary treatment causing costs to soar. The intent of the above commercial was to deceptively convey the impression that cancer patients had risen up and united in opposition to the proposed limitations but it was actually a fake group set up by a public relations firm. This example reflects the growing trend widely referred to as "Astrofurfing" in which fake, phony non-profit organizations are set up by segments of the medical industrial complex to lobby congress to further their own interests. Instead of being one of the legitimate patient advocacy and support organizations that actually represent the interest of patients, these groups represent the interests of the health care industry that benefit from what they are advocating. Astroturf organizations are increasing in number and are evident in all segments of society. They are particularly evident in health care including prostate cancer.

Most people don't fully understand what an Astroturf organization is and what it seeks to do. The primary purpose of such organizations is deception in that they pretend to be something they are not. Even though they are set-up as non-profit organizations, they are "front groups" shielding their corporate sponsors who are pursuing their own agendas. Unlike many real grass root organizations that have to struggle for funds, Astroturf organizations have almost unlimited funds. They use their money to hire highly talented employees to staff and run their fake groups. They are skilled at recruiting real patients who either volunteer or are paid a salary. Such groups are good at what they do and their websites reflect the best that money can buy. Using established legal, public relations, advertizing, marketing, research, and other consultants they engage in effective market analyses using focus groups to see what works and what does not work in terms of swaying the public to support their corporate agenda.

There is growing concern over the increasing number of Astroturf front groups masquerading as independent patient support groups. The confounding issue is that some of these groups DO provide valuable and helpful information and services. Most provide forums where patients can learn about their particular health problem and derive support from seeing how others have dealt with the same problem. Many of these groups started off being truly objective, independent organizations without any corporate agenda but were gradually usurped by segments of the medical-industrial complex. The problem is their deception in pretending to be independent grassroots non-profit patient organizations.

While some of Astroturf groups do provide valuable services, presenting themselves as grass root patient advocacy groups is highly disingenuous not only to the members who have joined the organization with a sincere desire to help a loved one or a family member but to the people influenced by their advocacy statements. Many of these organizations have been set up on a national basis with chapters in most of the states and have 'members' in excess of 100,000. When you encounter a slick cancer website with all of the latest improvements, look for a link to a section labeled "About Us." Click on this link and review the background of those managing the website. Also look at the Board of Directors. As you study this information you will likely see a number of individuals with close ties to the medical industrial complex. What you won't see is a statement indicating who is supporting the website.

A revealing article was published by Jeanne Lenzer in the March 2003 issue of the British Medical Journal stating "Us Too! International," one of the largest non-profit patient advocacy and support organizations in the world, received 95% of its funding from the pharmaceutical industry. The article went on to state that "The fact that certain 'grassroots' organizations have heavy funding from the drug industry may come as a surprise to much of the public, which has faith in the independence of non-profit organizations."[19]

It is important to keep in mind that not all non-profit patient advocacy and support groups are Astroturf organizations. A problematic sign is when such groups don't reveal their source of funding. Astroturf patient support and advocacy groups will continue to further the goals of their corporate sponsors. An example is their opposition to curtailing the routine use of PSA in screening healthy men. Some patient advocacy groups are joining in urging that the proposed policy not be followed and that the PSA still be used in routine screening. Some of these groups sincerely believe that the PSA screening should continue in its present format and have arrived at this decision independent of any outside influence or pressure. The problem is that when patient advocacy groups are largely funded by those who benefit financially from the continued use of the PSA for routine screening in healthy men, the issue of their objectivity being influenced by such funding arises.

Ray Moynihan, journalist, Iona Heath, general practitioner, and David Henry, professor of clinical pharmacology published a fascinating article on how patient advocacy groups are used to achieve the goals of the medical health industrial complex in the article titled "Selling sickness: the pharmaceutical industry and disease mongering." Published in the British Medical Journal in 2002 and cited from a National Cancer Institute linked website these authors stated: "Within many disease categories informal alliances have emerged, comprising drug company staff, doctors, and consumer groups. Ostensibly engaged in raising public awareness about under diagnosed and undertreated problems, these alliances tend to promote a view of their particular condition as widespread, serious, and treatable. Because these "disease awareness" campaigns are commonly linked to companies' marketing strategies, they operate to expand markets for new pharmaceutical products. Alternative approaches—emphasizing the self limiting or relatively benign natural history of a problem or the importance of personal coping strategies—are played down or ignored." [20]

Astroturfing can't survive in the light of day. It survives best when its true identify is hidden. A growing number of physicians, medical journals, and medical institutions have adopted the policy of requiring disclosure of any funding provided by any segment of the medical industrial industry. In an ideal world, patient advocacy and support groups funded by large health corporations would disclose their funding so that when they make public statements this fact can be taken into consideration. The problem is shining light on their funding destroys the purpose of their existence which is deception. Astroturf groups would not be very effective if they had to disclose who was operating and funding them.

At the time this book is being published a battle of monumental proportions was developing in the field of prostate cancer over the recommendations of the Task Force recommendations on the screening use of the PSA test in healthy men. On both sides respected health care specialists argue for or against the recommendations. If the task Force recommendations are followed (they were finalized on 5-22-12, see Chapter 12), there will be a significant reduction in active treatment of prostate cancer and a large number of men will be spared from harmful treatment that does not extend their life. There will also be a significant drop in income made by the prostate cancer industry which it does not want. But the Prostate Cancer Industry has its ace in the hole, the Astroturf groups it has set up across America. Among the loudest voices opposing the proposed changes will be their Astroturf groups. The money it invested in developing and funding these groups will pay off as they deceptively present themselves as legitimate grass root organizations set up by concerned patients. Like the fictitious example presented at the beginning of this section, a major marketing effort will swing into action as the prostate cancer industry uses their Astroturf organizations to urge the continued use of the PSA in screening healthy men.

Conclusion

Rough waters are ahead for many of you newly diagnosed with prostate cancer. On the face of it, following the recommendations of the urologist who diagnoses your prostate cancer seems to make sense. The problem is that powerful incentives have become associated with some types of treatments. Such treatments may generate significant financial gain for the urologist but it may also generate significant suffering from serious side effects that could have been avoided. Medical ethicists and regulatory agencies continue to try to address the abuses related to physician self-referral but it may be a long time before they make any headway. The issue of how best to use the PSA is less clear. Valid, well-intentioned views exist for and against its continued use in the screening of healthy men. As a prostate cancer survivor I see value in its use for screening but I also see the abuse in how it is used to steer men to treatment that may not be in their best interests. So that you will be better informed, when your urologist diagnoses prostate cancer and recommends surgery or IMRT he/she or an associate provide, ask if he/she has a financial investment in these devices used in such treatment. The bottom line is that the big money associated with the prostate cancer industry will likely succeed in preventing the task force recommendations minimizing the use of the PSA from being followed. Their Astroturf organizations will likely disseminate biased information designed to generate fear and uncertainty in men with prostate cancer with the goal being men demanding it from their physician.

The perilous nature of prostate cancer today has some people thinking of it as a national public health disaster. In such a situation you have to increase your knowledge of the various treatments and their side effects as well as seek a second opinion from an internist or medical oncologist. Every man newly diagnosed with prostate cancer needs to be aware of the five perils of the Prostate Cancer Industry.

The Five Perils of the Prostate Cancer Industry

Men newly diagnosed with prostate cancer face the following five perils from the Prostate Cancer Industry:

(1) The power from the huge amount of money generated by the current treatment of prostate cancer that leads many men into unnecessary overtreatment.

(2) Significant incentivizing of surgery and IMRT treatments, two treatments with high risks of side effects.

(3) The expanding practice of physician self referral to these two incentivized treatments.

(4) Major marketing efforts of prostate cancer treatment with high risks of side effects that are frequently misleading and discrediting of proton therapy and other less invasive treatments.

(5) Astroturf organizations operated and funded by segments of the medical industrial complex masquerading as spontaneous grass root patient groups.

Chapter Twelve

Why Prostate Cancer Treatment Is A National Health Disaster

"I never dreamt that my discovery 4 decades ago would lead to such a profit-driven public health disaster."1

Dr. Richard Ablin, Discussing
how the PSA is being used

Cures That Are Worse Than the Problem

The magnitude of the public health disaster resulting from how prostate cancer is treated can best be understood by the simple fact that most of its cures are worse than the problem of cancer. Let's look at the numbers. Around 240,000 men will be diagnosed with prostate cancer 2012, the year this book was published. At least 200,000 plus of these men will receive treatment. Over 160,000 of them will likely be steered into surgery or IMRT provided by either the urologist who diagnosed their cancer or by one of their associates. Of the approximately 160,000 men treated for prostate cancer in 2012, at least 50%, roughly 80,000+ men, will experience serious side effects that will significantly diminish the overall quality of their life. Many of these men could have survived their prostate cancer without such serious side effects. No matter how they are computed, the above numbers add up to a major public health disaster. It's that simple.

Don't be one of the above men.

The seriousness of the risks of adverse side effects from prostate cancer was actually confirmed on 5-22-12, the day this book was being set-up for publishing. On that day The U.S. Preventive

Services Task Force, the independent group of prevention and evidence-based medicine medical experts, finalized their recommendation that PSA screening results in over diagnosis of prostate cancer and unnecessary treatment that can leave men impotent and incontinent. I read their final recommendation in a report on News.Yahoo.com that stated "the task force concluded screening may only help one man in every 1,000 to avoid dying from prostate cancer. Up to five in 1,000 men will die within a month of prostate cancer surgery, the panel said, and between 10 and 70 per 1,000 men will suffer lifelong adverse effects, such as urinary incontinence, erectile dysfunction and bowel dysfunction."[2] The basic thrust of this book is consistent with their final recommendation.

I remain amazed at the number of men still electing to receive surgery for their prostate cancer. Urologist Bert Vorstman pulls no punches as he criticizes the use of surgery: "Currently, men concerned about possible prostate cancer will enter the unbelievable circus of prostate cancer evaluation and treatment where inaccuracies, subjectivity issues, misuse of investigational aids, shameful use of non-standard and self-serving definitions of success and complications in self-serving clinical studies as well as blatant conflicts of interest and financial incentives are pervasive. In addition, there is a common ploy by physicians for intentionally implying a sense of urgency and coercing an impulsive, uninformed, gullible and unsuspecting patient's decision for robotic surgery. This despicable process is coupled commonly with the practice of fear mongering and providing misleading information intentionally in order to manipulate a patient psychologically with the word "cancer" towards a high-risk, invasive and irreversible surgical treatment. In most educated circles, this would be called abuse."[3]

Solving the Prostate Cancer Conundrum

The Prostate Cancer Conundrum refers to the dilemma men diagnosed with prostate cancer face in the absence of a definitive test determining if their prostate cancer is the aggressive type that can kill them. They can either not receive treatment or run the risk of having a deadly form of cancer that could kill them or receive treatment they may not need that has serious side effects. There is a way to solve this conundrum.

1. Select Treatment with the Least Side Effects

The problem with the ongoing debate over the routine use of the PSA is that it is being framed incorrectly. The strongest arguments against its routine screening use is that prostate cancer treatments have the risks of producing serious side effects and treatment should be discouraged unless absolutely necessary. This argument is weakened by the availability of alternative treatments without the significant risk of serious side effects. One such treatment is proton therapy. The point of this book and many other similar books is to encourage men to consider proton therapy for the treatment of their prostate cancer. In selecting such treatments that have minimal side effects the arguments made by those opposing routine use of the PSA weaken.

The overwhelming majority of men newly diagnosed with prostate cancer have to decide on one of two options. One option is to not treat their prostate cancer and to engage in watchful waiting. If this is what they select they will be closely followed for any sign of their cancer becoming more advanced. The downside of this option is that it is not possible to determine if the type of cancer we develop is the serious type that could kill us. Thus, watchful waiting carries with it concern over not treating cancer that could be deadly. The other option is to treat their prostate cancer by selecting treatment with the risks of serious side effects such as surgery or IMRT. The good news is that the answer to the prostate cancer conundrum is, in my opinion, in selecting a minimally invasive treatment such as proton therapy. Doing this will not only allow you to treat your prostate cancer in case you have the type that could kill you, it also does not expose you to the risk of serious side effects. Dr. Vorstman passionately encourages men to consider non-invasive treatments of prostate cancer when he states: "Over the last few years, sophisticated advancements in several minimally invasive technologies such as cryoablation, radiation/proton, hifu and others have seriously questioned once more the very unfounded and controversial place of the heavy-handed, high-risk traditional surgical and robotic excision of prostate cancer. Time has made it quite clear that no amount of technology can circumvent the problems that necessarily result from the cutting out of your prostate." [3]

2. Indentifying Genetic Markers for Prostate Cancer - PCA3 gene

Another potential way of solving the prostate cancer conundrum is a promising new test for identifying men at risk of having aggressive prostate cancer involving analyzing urine for the presence of the PCA3 gene.[4] Molecular diagnostics has resulted in a specific test for identifying the urinary PCA3 gene found to be related to the presence of deadly, aggressive prostate cancer. This test can be a valuable alternative to the PSA Test in that it has greater ability to identify the risk of possessing deadly prostate cancer. If it becomes widely used as an alternative to the PSA, the goal of reducing the number of men referred for treatment with the risk of serious side effects can be achieved. If it does become widely used two consequences will occur: (1) fewer men will receive treatment they don't need and (2) the amount of money generated by unnecessary treatment will drastically reduce the profits of the prostate cancer industry. With this latter possibility in mind, don't be surprised if a crescendo of criticism of this new test develops. Any threat to the huge profits generated by the way prostate cancer is now treated will not be well received.

Conclusion

For those of you who have recently been diagnosed with prostate cancer, it is my hope that you will find this book helpful. Critics will point out the errors, omissions, and perhaps from their perspective, exaggerations in this book. I've tried to be accurate but readily admit my bias in favor of proton therapy. Concern over how the prostate cancer industry is currently operating has also influenced what is in this book. While critics may question some of the information I present, there is one fact that they can't challenge. That fact is my personal satisfaction in having gone through what turned out to be a surprisingly enjoyable treatment program with few if any side effects. I have no side effects whatsoever and continue to lead a full, productive life. I share these results with the vast majority of other men who have gone through proton therapy.

I am now at the end of my journey in prostate cancer. All I have left are continuing follow-up monitoring appointments that will likely go on in one fashion or another for another ten years. I know there are no guarantees in life and that a certain amount of risk is present in every prostate cancer treatment including proton therapy. I also know that not everyone going through surgery, IMRT, or other prostate cancer treatment will develop severe side effects. Many men go through these procedures with little difficulty and have few side effects. But the side effects for those who get them are so severe to make selecting one of these treatments a game of Russian roulette.

The problems of profit driven treatment described in this book are common throughout medicine and the field of health care. I readily admit that I do not fully understand these issues and simply look at them from the perspective of a patient. I can't help but wonder if a different, somehow better approach is needed in terms of how our health care is provided. Many of the problems described in this book come from the natural desire most of us have to increase our income. Surely there must be a better way for health care providers and institutions to increase their income without our suffering needlessly in the process. One possibility is my understanding of what physician Philip Caper recommended in 2009 when he advocated the elimination of the fee for service system and instead global budgets be adopted for hospitals with salaries and bonuses for doctors focused on maintaining health. This would remove the influence of fees for individual services on clinical decisions and would eliminate the single largest driver of exploding costs in American health care.[5] I hope I have accurately described Dr. Caper's view. Such an approach seems to make more sense than our current profit driven system.

I have returned to my life as it was before developing cancer. As you can tell by the tone and message of this book, I am quite happy with the treatment I received. I now look forward to enjoying the rest of my life free from any treatment side effects that would have lowered its overall quality. This is my first and last book on prostate cancer and the prostate cancer industry. I mention this fact in the hope that I don't become a target of the prostate cancer industry. It does happen. In my remaining years I have other priorities. First and foremost is spending time with my lovely grandchildren along with my family, and friends. I am also considering reforming the Diamondhead Regimental Brass Band, a military style community brass band I formed prior to developing prostate cancer. Then there is my hobby of restoring old military vehicles. My life is full and complete and will keep me busy and upon publication of this book I will leave prostate cancer and the prostate cancer industry behind me.

I hope this book will be helpful to those of you who are about to take the same journey I took. I urge those of you newly diagnosed with prostate cancer to exercise caution and seek second and third opinions from other medical specialties such as medical oncology or internal medicine and to study the various treatments paying careful attention to their side effects. Hopefully such an approach to your prostate cancer will bring you to a point at the end of your journey similar to one at which I have arrived.

I am not anti-urologist or anti-physician. I have had nothing but positive experiences with the urologists and other physicians I've encountered. I am, however pro patient and believe it is crucial for all of us to become better informed about any illness we may have and that we seek several opinions from independent physicians before agreeing to major treatment being recommended to us.

Yes, I've had my prostate cancer treated successfully by proton therapy and life for me is now good again. It's the same with the vast majority of patients I know who went through treatment with me.

Life can also be good for you.

Appendix A

Keeping It Up - Erectile Fitness Training

"Don't knock masturbation - its sex with someone I love"
Woody Allen

Joel Block, Ph.D. and Harold Dawley, Ph.D.

Joel Block, Ph.D

Joel is a psychologist practicing couple and sex therapy on Long Island, New York, where he has been honored with the Marriage and Family Therapist of the Year award. Board Certified in Couple Therapy, Dr. Block is a Senior Psychologist on the staff of North Shore-Long Island Jewish Health System where he supervised the hospital's Sexuality Center for 20 years. He is an Assistant Clinical Professor of Psychiatry at the Einstein College of Medicine. He is the author of numerous magazine articles and nineteen books, including *Sex Over 50*,[1] which is enjoying a second printing and Broken Promises, Mended Hearts[2], *Secrets of Better Sex*,[7] *The Art of the Quickie: Fast Sex, Fast Orgasm, Anytime, Anywhere*[4] and *She Comes First: 15 Ways to Save Your Relationship—without leaving the bedroom.*[5]

Why this Section was Written

When my colleague Harold Dawley asked me to join him in providing some information for this book on the importance of erectile fitness training I welcomed the opportunity. The two of us had just finished the book *The New Sexually Assertive Woman – A Guide for Women Seeking Good Sex*[6], coauthored with our colleague Victoria Zdrok, Ph.D. JD. Harold's role in our book is that of an expert on assertiveness while Joel's expertise is in sex therapy. After writing a book intended to help women achieve good sex, we concluded why not once again write material on helping men experience good sex by being able to maintain erectile fitness.

While the following information is intended for men who have completed treatment for prostate cancer, we believe that men in general will also find it helpful. Maintaining erectile fitness is important for men at any age and as men age it becomes even more important.

The Importance of Erectile Fitness

It can be quite distressing for men who had good erectile ability to discover that they have lost this ability after treatment for prostate cancer. Erection problems are common in adult men. In fact, almost all men experience occasional difficulty getting or maintaining an erection. In many cases, it is a temporary condition that will resolve with little or no treatment. In other cases, it can be an ongoing problem that can damage a man's self regard and harm his relationship with his partner, and thus requires treatment.

You have an erectile problem if you have difficulty getting or keeping an erection more than 25% of the time you engage in sexual relations. Many medical treatments for prostate cancer lead to ED with surgery having the greatest likelihood of producing it. The first fact to realize is that as we age many of our functions begin to decline.

One key function that can decline as men age is their ability to obtain and maintain an erection sufficient enough to complete sexual intercourse leading to orgasm. There is a corresponding decline in erectile function with 50% of men having experienced erectile problems by age 50. By age 70, this percentage goes up to 70% of men having had an ED experience. Vascular problems can occur that prevent blood from completely filling the spongy, tubular areas of the penis sufficiently to maintain an erection and is the most common physical basis for erectile problems. High blood pressure, diabetes, too much alcohol, and other problems can also be associated with erectile problems. Medications, especially some of those prescribed for cardiovascular issues, are another significant factor. Arousal problems can also lead to erectile problems. Men with low libido can also have difficulty maintaining an erection.

Our focus in this Section is primarily on the physical basis for erectile problems as those are the ones we think erectile fitness efforts will impact most significantly. We recommend erectile fitness training (EFT) for men with erectile organic (physical) problems and while it may not help all men, we believe it can be most helpful for men who had good erectile ability prior to prostate cancer treatment. We will also touch lightly on some of the psychological factors associated with erectile problems.

How does an Erection Occur?

Before going any further, let's check into Penis 101 and provide you with a description of how an erection works. Two chambers called the corpora cavernosa run the length of the penis (see Figure 1). A spongy tissue fills the chambers. A membrane, called the tunica albuginea, surrounds the corpora cavernosa. The spongy tissue contains smooth muscles, fibrous tissues, veins, and arteries. The urethra, which is the channel for urine and ejaculate, runs along the underside of the corpora cavernosa and is surrounded by the corpus spongiosum.

An erection begins with sensory or mental stimulation, or both. A man either thinks erotic thoughts or his penis is physically stimulated. Impulses from the brain and local nerves cause the muscles of the corpora cavernosa to relax, allowing blood to flow in through the arteries and fill the spaces. The blood creates pressure in the corpora cavernosa, making the penis expand much like air being pumped into a football makes it expand. A valve-like device at the base of the penis, the tunica albuginea, helps trap the blood in the corpora cavernosa, thereby sustaining the erection. After a man achieves orgasm or when sexual stimulation stops, the erection subsides when muscles in the penis contract to stop the inflow of blood and the valve-like device opens for blood outflow.

Figure 1. Arteries and veins of the penis

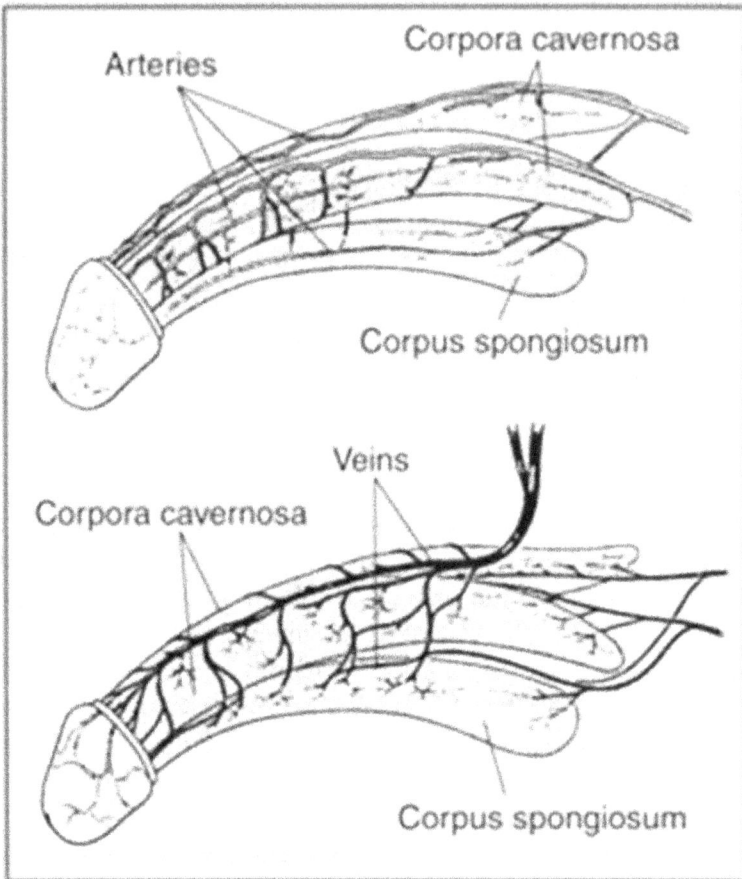

Reproduced from: National Kidney & Urologic Diseases Information Clearinghouse (NKUDIC) a service of the National Institute of Diabetes and Digestive and Kidney Diseases (NIDDK) National Institutes of Health (NIH)

Use It or Lose It

Like many aspects of the human body, the process of obtaining and maintaining an erection sufficient for satisfactory sexual intercourse is closely related to the frequency of this activity. Men who seldom obtain an erection and/or orgasm are at a significantly higher risk of developing ED than men who regularly do so. This risk applies both to men who have been treated for prostate cancer as well as to men in general.

The key factor in maintaining erectile fitness is the regular flow of blood to the arteries and veins in the penis. This blood brings needed oxygen and nutrients to vessels, tissue, and nerves in the penis. Think of this process as being similar to a plant that is regularly watered and fed that is doing well in comparison to a plant that is not regularly watered and fed that does not do well. When regular blood flow resulting in the engorgement of the penis does not happen, a man is at a higher risk of developing ED because the tissue inside the penis is not being nurtured. Similarly, woman who seldom engage in sexual intercourse are at risk of developing vaginal atrophy in which insertion of the penis into their vagina can be difficult and painful due to the withering away of the vagina from inaction.

For men to maintain good erectile fitness, they need to engage in regular sexual activity leading to orgasm two to three times a week. This means they engage in sexual intercourse, masturbation, or employ some other type of EFT to keep the oxygen and nutrients flowing into their penis.

The good news is that regular sexual activity in which you maintain an erection leading to orgasm at least two to three times week will help to maintain your erectile fitness. The bad news is that the absence of such regular sexual activity can significantly increase the odds of developing erectile dysfunction. We all are aware of the advantages of regular physical exercise being correlated with good health in that the more we engage in regular physical activity such as walking or other exercise, the better our health. It is the same with maintaining erectile fitness.

Lifestyle Factors Related To ED

Since an erection is a cardio-vascular event, by far the most common factor leading to ED in men is a diminished cardiovascular system related to poor eating habits, sedentary life style, stress and being overweight. Being on certain medications, and having had some types of medical treatment can also lead to ED.

The aging process, if accompanied by arterioscleroses, results in the gradual accumulation of plaque on the walls of blood vessels that in turn restricts the flow of blood in the penis. In this process there is a gradual restriction that occurs in blood vessels leading to various organs. Some medical experts state that erectile problems are a precursor to heart disease and indicate an impaired cardiovascular system. When reduced blood flow leading to the heart occurs it is identified as coronary artery disease. Secondary to that is likely to be reduced blood flow to the penis and consequent erectile problems.

When adequate blood is prevented from reaching the heart there is the increased risk of a heart attack. When a blockage is so great that insufficient blood reaches the heart, part of the heart is damaged. The same process occurs with erections in men. Men, who have maintained a healthy lifestyle by avoiding fattening foods, have an adequate level of physical fitness, minimize stress, and do not use tobacco products or abuse drugs and alcohol are less likely to experience ED. This is the reason why men who enter treatment for prostate cancer who have good erectile fitness prior to treatment will likely have adequate erectile fitness after treatment.

Psychological Factors Related To Erectile Problems

Some men experience anxiety in anticipation of sexual relations. This anxiety can grow as they fear they will not perform well by not being able to maintain an erection. A self-fulfilling prophecy can occur in which men who experience this performance anxiety actually do have difficulty maintaining an erection. The anxiety they experience is the body's "fight or flight" adaptation that throws off adrenaline and drives blood from the penis into large muscles, like legs. The consequence is a flaccid penis. Reducing their level of anxiety so that normal arousal can occur can solve this problem. (See Dr. Block's Wellness Program, www.MindoverED.com) In addition to performance anxiety some other men have lowered libido in which their sexual arousal is reduced. Men who are taking hormone suppressant treatment in which testosterone is suppressed will see a loss in their libido. Still other men struggle with more complicated sexual or intimacy issues that interfere with their sexual functioning.

Erectile Dysfunction Following Treatment for Prostate Cancer

When men receive treatment for prostate cancer, the odds of their experiencing erectile problems go up greatly. Surgery results in a high percentage of erectile problems and many times there is little that can be done for it.

The benefits of conventional IMRT photon radiation and proton therapy are that these procedures have a significantly lower risk of erectile problems. But because the risk of such problems go up as men age and the fact that most men who receive such treatment for prostate cancer tend to be older, erectile fitness training can help to minimize the risk of erectile problems. It needs to be noted that in the context of prostate cancer treatment this discussion of erectile fitness training is directed to men who had relatively good erectile fitness prior to treatment for prostate cancer.

For those of you who want to be able to engage in sexual intercourse with your wife or significant other following radiation treatment for prostate cancer, there is hope. One of the problems commonly experienced following radiation treatment for prostate cancer is retrograde or limited ejaculation. For some men this is not a serious problem. For other men the feeling of ejaculating into their wife during sexual intercourse is a very desirable part of their sex life. These men want to maintain this ability to ejaculate if at all possible.

The urologist Dr. Bert Vorstman believes that some men can improve their ability to ejaculate more during sex.[11] (Personal Communication to author Harold Dawley). The key aspect for minimizing the risk of ED following treatment for prostate cancer in men who had good erectile functioning prior to treatment seems to be regular sexual activity leading to orgasm.

And that brings us to erectile fitness training.

Erectile Fitness Training

What is Erectile Fitness Training

Erectile fitness training is the process in which a man engages in sexual activity that involves obtaining and maintaining an erection leading to orgasm two to three times a week. It is based on the concept that erectile fitness can be enhanced by regular erectile exercises. These exercises involve sexual intercourse, oral sex (fellatio) or manual manipulation of the penis by your partner. When a partner is not available or is not willing, erectile fitness training also involves the use of masturbation. Various products and devices are available to assist you in your erectile fitness training. Like any fitness program it begins with having the right attitude. You thus need to realize the importance of erectile fitness in maintaining a good relationship with your wife or partner as well as maintaining a positive self-image. There is no reason guilt or shame has to be associated with this health-enhancing program.

Follow the Doctor's Advice - There's No Room for Guilt in Maintaining Your Erectile Fitness

When we wrote the book *The New Sexually Assertive Woman – A Guide for Women Seeking Good Sex*, one of the major problems we addressed was the pervasive sense of guilt many women have associated with taking an active role in sex. The "good girl stereotype" is common and holds many women back from being active in sex.

The reality is that only 40% of women achieve orgasm on a regular basis. The solution is for women who are not experiencing good sex is to become sexually assertive and to direct their man into doing what he needs to do for her to achieve satisfactory sex leading to a full orgasm. But to do this they have to overcome guilt that has been associated with the good girl stereotype. It is the same with men seeking to maintain the ability to engage in satisfactory sexual intercourse with their wife. They have to overcome any guilt they may have with engaging in erectile fitness training activity.

Incorrect and Harmful Beliefs about Masturbation

Even in contemporary society we never cease to be amazed by the number of men and women we encounter who believe that masturbation is not only morally wrong but that it can be harmful. We certainly respect the right of people to hold whatever religious beliefs they wish. But when such beliefs conflict with the facts it is important that they be corrected.

Believing that masturbation can make you blind, turn you into a sex pervert, or lead to ED is irrational in that there is no factual basis for such beliefs. While anything in excess could be problematic, we think that the regular act of masturbation as we describe it in this chapter can be helpful to men seeking to maintain erectile fitness.

Masturbation is an important part of EFT. The penis works best in terms of getting hard and staying hard during just about any type of sexual activity. Just as health experts agree that regular physical exercise is important part of maintaining good health, regular exercising of the penis is good for your erectile fitness. "Beating off, jacking off, self-abuse" are only a few of the negative terms used to describe the health enhancing activity of masturbation. Masturbation is practiced universally in every culture and society. For many young men masturbation is their major outlet for sexual release. Continuing to engage in masturbation before, during, and after treatment for prostate cancer is one of the best steps men can take to increase their chances of maintaining their erectile fitness.

A growing number of sex therapists and other health experts are encouraging men to engage in regular sexual activity as a way of maintaining their erectile ability. It should be pointed out that if a man has a willing partner, sexual intercourse can be engaged in instead of masturbation. If no partner is available then masturbation needs to be used for the EFT. Whatever a man does he must free himself from guilt associated with regular or occasional masturbation. It is, after all, what the doctors have ordered.

The Importance of First Satisfying Your Partner

Good sex occurs when both parties find it enjoyable and satisfying. It does not work when one party has all of the fun while the other does all of the work. Even though you may have had treatment for prostate cancer and need regular sexual stimulation this need is no justification for a selfish attitude of expecting your partner to pleasure you while you lay back and do nothing for her.

Your partner has sexual needs as well that also must be met. All too often we have seen such a lopsided sexual relationship can lead to a breakup of the relationship or marriage. Bad sex for a woman is when she does not achieve orgasm on a regular basis during sex with her man and that is not good for the relationship.

You are encouraged to satisfy your partner first before you achieve your satisfaction. The reason for this is simple - it can be difficult to work up the motivation to pleasure your woman after you have had an orgasm. It is certainly possible that some men are able to go on and pleasure their woman to satisfaction after they have achieved orgasm but the odds are great that when it happens more often than not the woman is going to be shortchanged.

The more you satisfy your wife or partner the greater likelihood she will be a willing partner in helping you maintain your erectile fitness.

Getting It Up

Erectile fitness training (EFT) starts with obtaining and maintaining an erection. For those of you who have an understanding partner this is an activity in which both of you can engage. If your wife or partner is unwilling to participate in sexual activity two to three times a week, you can visualize having sex with her to obtain an erection. Should visualizing scenes of having sex with your woman not be sufficient there are erotic images available on the Internet.

Viewing sexually erotic photos or videos is a common way for men to obtain an erection. A man can be aroused sexually by imagining having sex with his partner. For those of you who need additional visual erotic stimulation viewing photos or video of men and women engaging in sex can also be helpful in obtaining an erection. It is widely acknowledged that the most viewed imagery on the Internet is pornography.

More money is made from pornography websites than the combined income generated by the top five software/Internet companies such as Microsoft, Google, Amazon, EBay and Yahoo. Internet pornography is big business.

Orgasm

Once you have satisfied your partner sexually the next step is for you to achieve orgasm. Getting fully aroused with a firm erection is the first step in experiencing orgasm. Once your penis is firm, you can engage in sexual intercourse and hopefully have an orgasm. Even if you do not achieve an orgasm, sexual intercourse will still be good for your erectile fitness. Try to engage in such sexual activity two to three times per week. For men whose partner is not inclined to engage in regular sex two or three times a week they must then become sexually aroused in other ways. The logical method is masturbation.

The standard joke about masturbation is that 99% of men do and 1% lie about not doing it. The instinctual urge to procreate is so strong that men seek to release this urge by engaging in masturbation. We don't need to describe to you how to masturbate but what we do need to do is to encourage you to do so two or three times a week or have sex with your partner two or three times a week—or some combination of both. The key factor is obtaining an erection and orgasm. If it has to be done by masturbating to orgasm, then that is what you have to do. Thinking erotic thoughts or viewing erotic stimuli along with physical stimulation of your penis can bring it to an erection or semi-erection. Every time your penis becomes erect or semi-erect is good for you in terms of erectile fitness. If masturbation is the only way to bring your penis to erection, go for it. The key element of erectile fitness training is bringing your penis to erection so that the health enhancing blood and nutrients can reach the tissues and nerves in your penis.

Shooting Blanks – Retrograde Ejaculation
Harold's Experience

Somewhere around halfway through my treatment I began to notice that my orgasms during sex were dry. They were pleasurable but strange types of orgasms having a slight tinge of pain. In talking with other patients I quickly discovered they were also having the same experience. After being made aware of the importance of regular sexual activity I began ongoing erectile fitness training. I eventually reached the point at around seven months post treatment when I began having ejaculations in which I discharged more fluid. Over time the amount of fluid discharged increased and as it did, so did the amount of my pleasure. As I reflect back on this experience what comes to my mind is the expression, "You have to learn to crawl before you can learn to walk."

For most men who have gone through prostate cancer treatment, orgasm will culminate in a dry ejaculation, what is referred to as "retrograde ejaculation" or, as the patients call it, "shooting blanks." I recently came upon a blog where men shared their sexual problems following prostate cancer treatment. One man unabashedly wrote in colorful terms about his previous enjoyment in experiencing a full ejaculation. Describing his past ejaculatory experiences like a "rocket blasting off," he stated that the dry orgasms he was experiencing were quite a disappointment. There is regrettably little research on erectile fitness training following prostate cancer treatment. But based on anecdotal information from patients I've talked with along with discussions with urologists who have treated such men, it does appear that it is possible for some men to once again acquire the ability to actually ejaculate. With consistent erectile fitness training some men will find that they can eventually ejaculate an increasing amount of fluid. With this increased ejaculation, their sexual pleasure also increases.

Priming the Pump – Increasing Your Ejaculate

Most men find the process of ejaculation one of the most enjoyable parts of sexual intercourse. During sexual intercourse the excitement grows in intensity and reaches its highpoint during the ejaculatory process. When the amount of ejaculatory fluid is minimal, the enjoyment for many men is decreased. Even a slight increase in the ejaculation can increase a man's sexual pleasure.

There is a way men can increase the amount of fluid they ejaculate. We call it priming the pump and while it may seem somewhat crude to use this term it does describe the process we recommend. If you want to increase the amount of fluid you ejaculate, go ahead and engage in sexual activity bringing you close to the point of orgasm and then stop. Let the feeling subside. If you are in the middle of satisfying your wife or partner, go ahead and bring her to satisfaction.

Then go back to your stimulating activity with your partner; bring yourself to full arousal and again approach the point of almost experiencing an orgasm. Then stop your sexual activity. Let the feeling subside and once again engage in sexual activity and continue to orgasm. What you will find when you engage in this start and stop sexual arousal is that a fair amount of fluid will build up each time you get aroused. When you finally complete sex you will then ejaculate more fluid and your sexual pleasure increases.

Sex Aids to Facilitate Erection and Orgasm

Just as men and women are uncomfortable talking about wearing pads or diapers when they are incontinent, some men are uncomfortable about using mechanical aids to help them obtain and maintain their erectile ability. Fortunately, there are a number of products and devices that can provide such help to men and their use is becoming more common among men who have had prostate cancer and other health issues.

Lubricating Fluid

Lubricating fluids in either a liquid or ointment form are available that can not only lubricate the penis during its insertion into the vagina but can enhance pleasure during masturbation either by the man or his woman.

Vibrators

Long a standard device in sex therapy for women, vibrators can also be helpful for men. There are even vibrators shaped like an artificial vagina that can facilitate a man achieving orgasm during masturbation. One device, the Penisator, can actually be attached to the penis. Once attached to a limp penis, it can quickly bring it back alive and get it to full erection.

Sex Toys

A variety of sex toys are available on the Internet. You may not realize it but a booming business exists in the development, manufacture, and marketing of sex toys. Men can use these sex toys when they engage in masturbation or sexual activity with their wife or partner. Don't be shocked as we describe some of the more popular sex toys that are available to you. There are masturbatory sleeves that slide over the entire length of the penis, blow job imitators that mimic fellatio, artificial vaginas, and full size dolls with artificial vaginas build into to them.

Oral ED Drugs That Help Maintain Erections

For some of you erectile fitness training alone may not be enough for you to be able to engage in sexual intercourse with your wife or partner. Presented next are a variety of aids that can assist in allowing you to engage in more satisfying sexual intercourse. They begin with the use of orally administered drugs intended to treat ED.

There are three main drugs used in treating ED. They are Viagra, Levitra, and Cialis.

Sildenafil, the generic name for Viagra was developed by a group of scientists working for Pfizer. First studied as a possible treatment for high blood pressure and angina (heart pain), early research failed to demonstrate help for these problems. What they did discover were side effects of increased ability for a man to maintain a strong erection. Viagra was subsequently patented on March 1998 and quickly became a success with annual sales reaching close to $200 million dollars by 2008. Shortly thereafter, additional ED drugs appeared with the two leading contenders to Viagra being Cialis and Levitra. These drugs work by increasing the flow of blood into the penis in conjunction with erotic imagery and/or physical stimulation of the penis sufficiently for a man to successfully engage in sexual intercourse.

Viagra, Levitra, and cialis all belong to a drug class indentified as phosphodiesterase-5 (PDE-5) inhibitors. They work by allowing the blood vessels in the penis to relax sufficiently enough to allow blood to flow into the penis. When this increased blood flow is coupled with sexual arousal, an erection develops. All three of these drugs increase the ability to obtain and maintain an erection around 20 minutes after being taken. One big difference is that Viagra and Levitra remain effective for four to six hours while Cialis can remain effective for up to 36 hours.

Viagra (sildenafil)

Viagra remains the most popular ED drug in terms of sales. For most men it works in less than an hour allowing men to obtain a firm erection for a four hour period. It is important to note that an erection not be consistently active for this period of time because it could be harmful. The four-hour period simply means that a man has the increased ability to obtain an erection during this duration.

Levitra (vardenafil)

Levitra is a drug similar to Viagra in that it also has the ability to facilitate a firm erection in men who are sexually stimulated. Levitra works in the same way as Viagra with similar side effects and interactions. It is not as long-lasting as Cialis.

Cialis (tadalafil)

Cialis works in the same way as Viagra and Levitra but offers two important benefits, a 36-hour window of opportunity for intimacy and the ability to take the tablet on an empty stomach or with a meal. Cialis is becoming popular with men because its effects last so long. This increased time period means that sex can be more spontaneous.

Side Effects of Oral ED Drugs

Most ED drugs have similar side effects. The most common side effects include headaches, slight blurring of vision, and upset stomach, and are similar for all three drugs. Some men find they can reduce these side effects by using a smaller dosage of the drug and still be able to maintain an erection. Some risks of side effects are more serious. Indeed, although not common, there have been deaths reported.

Sometimes a man may find that one of these drugs works just as well at a smaller-than-usual dose with less risk of side effects and still experiences the result he wants. Viagra, Levitra, and Cialis can lead to dangerous drug interactions when men with heart disease are taking nitrates like nitroglycerine or isosorbide (Isordil, Ismo, Imdur).

Other Ways of Taking ED Drugs

Injections into penis: ED erection-inducing agents include injection and insertion of pellets into the penis. One procedure involves injecting drugs such alprostadil (Caverject) into the shaft of the penis that relax the penile blood vessels and allow for engorgement of blood into the penis. Once injected, the chemicals facilitate the attainment of erection coupled with sexual arousal.

Inserting pellets into urethra: a drug containing alprostadil is available in a pellet form (Muse) that can be inserted into the urethra. Once inserted the chemical is released and has a similar reaction in terms of facilitating the relaxation of blood vessels in the penis to allow blood flow to increase when sexually aroused.

The above methods have become less popular since the increasing availability of oral drugs. For a small minority of men they seem to work well.

Penile Constriction Devices

There are other ways in which you can obtain and maintain an erection other then medications. One common approach is a penile constriction device that is known as a vacuum constriction device (VCD). This device employs an acrylic cylinder that is slipped over the penis. There is a pump attached to the cylinder operated by hand or battery that then pumps out air creating a vacuum that draws blood into the penis causing it to swell and produce an erection. A strong rubber ring previously attached to the vacuum cylinder is then slid down the shaft of the penis to its base where it then traps the blood that has been drawn into the penis. The vacuum is then released from the penis and the external pump is removed. With the penis now erect you can now begin intercourse. The restraining ring can safely be left on the base of the penis for up to 30 minutes before it must be removed. After completion of sexual intercourse the constriction ring is slid off the lubricated penis and the blood flows out ending the erection.

Over 50% of men are satisfied with the results of using vacuum constriction devices, as they are able to produce an erection and engage in sexual intercourse. The constriction ring tends to reduce the amount of ejaculatory fluid released during orgasm. A black and blue bruise may be evident at the base of the penis where the ring was in place. Over time some men report that their level of satisfaction in using such devices tends to decrease. A certain amount of caution must be exercised in using such devices by ensuring they contain a "quick release" that promptly releases the vacuum. Possible injuries to the penis may occur if the vacuum is not released in a timely manner.

The price range for VCD's range from $300 to $600 and there are a number of good ones on the market. Your health insurance may cover part of the cost of purchasing one.

Penile Implants

A penile implant is the insertion into the penis of a either a semi-rigid device or an inflatable device a man can use to produce an erection sufficient for sexual intercourse. A semi-rigid device involves the insertion of a flexible cylinder into the penis that provides enough firmness for sexual intercourse. When a man is ready for sexual intercourse he reaches down and bends his penis into position to permit insertion into the vagina of his partner. A major drawback of the semi-rigid device is that their insertion into the penis destroys the normal process of obtaining an erection. In other words, a man will no longer be able to get an erection through normal blood flow. With inflatable devices two cylinders are also inserted into the penis along with a supply of saline in the abdomen. A release is placed in the scrotum for bringing the fluid into the tubes, simulating blood flow and creating an erection. Another mechanism is also placed in the scrotum to bring the fluid out of the tubes ending the erection with the penis returning to a flaccid state.

A major disadvantage of penile implants is the destruction of the normal erectile mechanism.

Conclusion - Getting and Staying in Shape Sexually

We have presented a wide array of options for those of you who have either gone through treatment for prostate cancer or are contemplating it. Your first step is to carefully study the risk of developing serious sexual side effects present with different treatments. As indicated throughout this book, all prostate cancer treatments work equally well and primarily differ in terms of the side effects.

The greatest risk of serious side effects occurs in surgery, which is also the treatment most men are encouraged to select. Proton therapy has the least risk of side effects and has a low risk of developing sexual problems after treatment.

Regardless of your treatment, you will find it helpful to engage in erectile fitness training prior to starting your treatment and maintain it throughout treatment and afterwards as well. Some of you will find it helpful to take ED drugs and will need to work closely with your physician to find the one best for you. For more stubborn cases of ED other options have also been presented.

The bottom line is that like any exercise, repetition and consistency are important. Any man wishing to engage in EFT will find it helpful to get into the routine of becoming sexually aroused and either engaging in sex with his partner or masturbating to orgasm several times a week.

Reference Notes

1. Joel Block, *Sex Over Fifty*, Penguin Group, Paperback, 2008.
2. Joel Block, *Broken Promises, Mended Hearts : Maintaining Trust in Love Relationships*, McGraw-Hill, 2001.
3. Joel Block, *Secrets of Better Sex: A Noted Sex Therapist Reveals His Secrets to Passionate Sexual Fulfillment* by Joel D. Block, Prentice Hall Press, 2001.
4. Joel Block, *Art of the Quickie, Fast Sex, Fast Orgasm, Sex Anytime, Anywhere*, Quiver, 2006.
5. Joel Block & Kimberly Newman, *She Comes First: 15 Ways To Save Your Relationship*, Adams Media, 2009.
6. Victoria Zdrok, Joel Block, & Harold Dawley, *The New Sexually Assertive Woman*, in press.
7. Albert Vorstman, Personal Communication to Harold Dawley

Appendix B

Facilitated Patient Support –

A Valuable Part of Medical Treatment

"Woe to he who is alone when he falleth, for he have not another to help him up."

The Bible

Going Through Treatment with Friends

Facilitated Patient Support describes the facilitation of the health enhancing effects of going through treatment with friends. When we go through treatment, particularly prolonged treatment such as is common in many types of cancer, doing so with friends generates a powerful health enhancer called social support. Social support can occur naturally among patients going through a treatment program together that not only makes the experience more positive but can increase its effectiveness as well. Medicine has long recognized the importance of a caring and compassionate attitude among physicians as referenced by the long awareness of the importance of a good bedside manner. Social support from other patients can be an even more important component to health treatment. Long a neglected part of heath care, support from going through treatment with friends can be a powerful health enhancer.

Up until now, patient support occurs naturally as patients make friends with each other. Its occurrence is incidental and it is a matter of chance whether or not this powerful factor is a part of treatment. If the scheduling of treatment coincidentally arranges for the same patients to receive treatment at the same time and place, then the chances are that they will develop supportive social relationships with one another similar to the warrior bond I experienced at the proton therapy center. But it is generally a happenchance occurrence of unplanned or uncoordinated events that fortuitously results in the development of the health enhancing social support.

But what if various treatment programs took deliberate steps in treatment planning to ensure that the factors are present to allow this therapeutic modality to occur?

It took many years before health care researchers recognized the importance of social support in health care. It was so obvious that it was overlooked even though healthcare providers have long known that patients who had loving and caring wives and other close relationships did significantly better than those lacking such meaningful relationships. It was a matter of observing two factors that seemed to correlate with each other such as people who were not significantly overweight tended to do better following many different types of health care treatments than people who were overweight. Dieticians now routinely work with many patients who are overweight as they are taught the importance of healthy eating and exercise. While we now know that the presence of good social support and maintaining normal weight contributes to treatment success, it took many years before their importance was recognized. Social workers, psychologists, and other mental health professionals now help medical patients improve their level of social support by encouraging marriage counseling to mend troubled marriages. But there is another adjunctive factor that can significantly contribute to the success of various health care treatments and that is, when feasible, ensuring that as patients go through the same treatment together, deliberate efforts are made to increase their chances of bonding together.

For many years, physicians and other health care providers have noted that when patients went through protracted treatments such as the delivery of radiation in small doses to kill cancer, they tended to naturally bond with one another. The phenomenon of propinquity and proximity would kick in and as these patients started to get to know each other, they developed strong supportive relationships. As this social support developed, they benefited from it in terms of experiencing a greater level of life satisfaction and a lowering of anxiety associated with their specific health problem and its treatment. But for the most part, the development of such support remained a chance byproduct of the process of scheduling treatment.

It's seems to be a different story at the MD Anderson Proton Therapy Center and Loma Linda Proton treatment. Their patients seem to bond together and derive support from each other. At Loma Linda, The Brotherhood of the Balloon, a patient support group founded by Bob Marckini, ProtonBob.com, also provides support and encouragement to men going through treatment for prostate cancer. At the Proton Therapy Center at MD Anderson ProtonPals, an organization of former proton therapy patients run by former prostate cancer patient Joe Landry, provides support and organizes regular weekly dinners fostering an ongoing sense of social bonding among them.

Other medical and treatment centers are encouraged to incorporate into their patient's treatment planning ways in which all of the patients will go through treatment with the same group of other patients so that social bonding is facilitated. Instead of looking at a treatment schedule that works best for the medical staff or for the health care facility, treatment should be scheduled to foster the naturally occurring social support that can develop among people going through protracted treatment together. This means that a priority effort should be made to ensure that patients keep the same schedule as they progress through treatment. The big pay off for the medical center providing the treatment is a happier more relaxed patient population who experience the benefits of social support along with the actual medical treatment they receive.

When men and women join the military they go through basic training with a group of other men and women. Formed into a platoon or some other military organization they get to know each other as they go through training together. As expected, strong friendship bonds develop among many of them. A similar approach could easily be used in providing some types of medical treatment. For any medical condition in which a large number of treatments spaced over time are required, forming patients together so that they start treatment at the same time and progress through it together can foster the social camaraderie and bonding that normally occurs in such settings. As each group of patients is formed the group could be identified in some special way such as "The Summer Class of 2011." Such a designation can also facilitate bonding and increase the feeling of being a member of a unique group.

My initial impression from going through the Proton Therapy Center at MD Anderson was that the social bonding that occurs there is an unintentional by-product of the treatment. I did not see any specific efforts to keep the same group of men together or any other deliberate effort to foster social bonding and camaraderie. Scheduling seemed to be more attuned to providing as much treatment to as many men as possible. Little advance planning was evident in terms of offering permanent time slots to men registering for treatment. Not once did anyone mention or describe the importance of social bonding. What little awareness of the importance of social bonding seemed to come from a few staff members. One nurse practitioner did appear to realize its importance and was very active in encouraging the weekly dinners. Tai Lee was the only staff member I encountered that appeared to have any awareness of the importance of social bonding and camaraderie. She took an active role in finding patients to coordinate the weekly dinners and frequently attended them herself. On at least one occasion, several Japanese medical students who were briefly working at the Proton Therapy Center also attended one of the dinner meetings. Credit goes to Tai Lee for helping to facilitate patient support at the Proton Therapy Center..

Since my completion of treatment the Proton Therapy Center, it has added a "Patient Facilitator" or some similar title, to facilitate patients' interactions and bonding. Long a leader in health care, M.D. Anderson's Proton Therapy Center is once again taking a lead in the direct facilitation of patient support.

Fellowship Coordinators to Facilitate Patient Bonding

My wife and I have been on countless cruises. One of the procedures used on virtually all cruise ships is the assignment of staff that has specific responsibility for encouraging people on the ship to interact with each other. Anyone who has taken a cruise will know what I am describing. There are all kinds of silly games designed for the people on the ship to get to know each other. Health care facilities could employ a similar procedure in which staff members would have specific responsibility for fostering camaraderie among patients going through a treatment program together. Such a staff member could do what Tai Lee does at the Proton Therapy Center and organize social events for the patients. I am hopeful that the "Patient facilitator" recently added to the proton therapy center will fill this role. Ample opportunities exist for facilitating such social activities whenever a group of patients are going through a protracted treatment program together.

Facilitating Patient Support Must Be Viewed an Important Component of Treatment

To tap into the valuable social camaraderie and the resultant social support it provides, leaders of medical centers that provide protracted treatment to groups of patients need to recognize the value of facilitating patient support. This means that a coordinated effort is required in which scheduling of treatment is done to facilitate the development of patient support. Staff members need to be assigned with specific responsibility for arranging social events that encourage social bonding among patients. It is only by such coordinated efforts that medical centers can be assured that they tap into the powerful social support from patient bonding.

To better understand the value of patient support, I conducted a survey among a group of patients who went through proton therapy with me. The results of this survey are presented next.

Patient Survey Results

Overview of Results

It was only as an afterthought that I decided to survey patients in terms of the importance they placed on the interaction and support with other patients with whom they went through treatment. I had already sent out the survey on how patients see their urologist discussed earlier and had not planned on doing any additional surveys. Consequently the response rate to this survey was disappointingly low. Enough patients did respond to give some indication as to how they felt about the social interaction with other patients. These results are presented next followed by the actual survey.

This survey began with the simple question "Did you make some good friends during your proton therapy treatment?" On this question every respondent answered "yes", indicating that they did make some good friends during their treatment. The next question dealt with their perceived importance of interacting and socializing with other patients. A surprising 79% reported that it was an important part of their treatment. When asked if laughing and joking with the other patients helped to reduce their fear and anxiety, 92% of the patients reported that it did help to reduce their fear and anxiety. Only one patient reported that the opportunity to laugh and joke with other patients did not play an important role in reducing his fear and anxiety. Seventy-five percent of the patients reported "Very much so" to having looked forward each day to talking with the other men going through treatment with them with the remaining 25% of the patients reporting "Yes, somewhat so.". When asked specifically about their participation in the weekly dinners, 61% reported that they went to some of them.

In terms of the social camaraderie and support that developed among them being the result of a deliberate policy on the part of the Proton Therapy Center, only 15 % of the patients believed it was a deliberate policy. When asked if they believed camaraderie and support from socializing with other patients going through proton therapy was important enough to make it a formal part of treatment almost 70% (69.2%) believed it was important enough to be a formal part of the treatment.

Some surprising results were evident in question number eight in which the patients ranked what they felt were the most important aspects of their treatment. The aspect "Going through treatment with many of the same patients" tied with "Your physician" in terms of what they felt was the most important part of the treatment. The two next highest ranked aspects of treatment were "Interacting with other patients" and "The opportunity to joke about the treatment."

From my standpoint one of the most important questions on this survey was number 10 which asked "Do you think treatment centers such as the Proton Therapy Center that provide daily treatment for a protracted period of time should actively facilitate social interaction among its patients?" A resounding 76.9% of the patients responded, "yes" indicating that they believed the mutual support they experienced from other patients was important enough to be actively facilitated. The next question dealt with how treatment centers could facilitate social support among its patients. Of the five ways of facilitating such support two were ranked highest. They are "Keeping the same appointment time to facilitate getting to know the other patients in that time slot" and "Distributing a list of names and phone numbers to all patients and encouraging them to contact each other."

Constant Contact Survey Results

Survey Name: May 30 2011 Survey
Response Status: Partial & Completed
Filter: None
7/18/2011 9:25 AM CDT

1. Did you make some good friends during your proton therapy treatment?

Number of responses, Percentage of responses
Yes: 13, 100.0%
No: 0,   0.0%
Total: 13 (81.2%)
Specific Comments

"I am convinced that the friendship and fellowship formed in the Men's Dressing Room just outside of Gantry 3, is integral in the healing process. We were allowed to explore our feelings, share our thoughts with others and most important of all LAUGH!"

"Lots of chit-chat friends." "Perhaps, it may be appropriate to say many new good acquaintances whom I enjoyed sharing the experience and information whom we may or may not see again." "I'd say I made some friends. I'll probably follow-up with an e-mail at a later date to see how they are doing."

"Probably more like some good acquaintances."

2. How important were the opportunities you had to interact and socialize with the other patients you met during treatment?

Number of responses, Percentage of responses
Most important: 2, 15.3%
Somewhat Important: 7, 53.8%
Not crucial: 4, 30.7%
Not important: 0, 0.0%
Specific Comments

"Have felt that the proper medical treatment, diet and lifestyle, and support to be three important keys to recovery." "I worked in Houston and lived just west of the city during my treatment. Therefore I was somewhat loathe to return to the city in the evening after going home from work."

"I was a local resident of Houston and worked during my treatment period. As a result, I didn't take advantage of the opportunities to socialize with the other patients."

3. Did laughing and joking with the other patients help to reduce your fear and anxiety with having prostate cancer?

Number of responses, Percentage of responses

Yes, very important role: 9, 56.2%

Yes, it helped somewhat: 6, 37.5%

No, not a factor: 1, 6.2%

Specific Comments

"Eliminated any thought of stress or fear. Had no anxiety because of my faith in God and faith in the Proton Therapy Center's professionalism, staff, and their knowledge of how to deliver the treatment tailored for my situation." "I don't think at this point I had any fear of having prostate cancer. It did help relieve my anxiety with the treatments."

4. Did you look forward each day to talking with the other men who were going through treatment with you?

Number of responses, Percentage of responses

Yes, very much so: 11, 73.3%

Yes, Somewhat so: 4, 26.6%

No,0, 0.0%

Specific Comments

"The atmosphere was fun, invigorating, and uplifting. Laughter is key in recovery...no heavy heart here..."

5. Did you participate in the weekly patient dinners at different restaurants?

Number of responses, Percentage of responses

Yes, every one I could: 5, 31.2%

Yes, I went to some: 4, 25%

No, schedule conflict: 1, 6.2%

No, not interested: 6, 37.5%

Specific Comments

"Wife sick during my treatment, went home to be with her." "I live in Houston and working. I was tired after work to participate." "The patient dinners were missed only because attending required an additional 3 hrs of driving to and from Houston another day of the week. I know that I missed good fellowship." "I would have had to stay around after work or drive back into Houston to attend the dinners. I chose to do neither."

6. Do you think the Proton Therapy Center has an established policy (other than the weekly dinners) to encourage the patients to make friends with one another?

Number of responses, Percentage of responses

Yes, part of the plan: 3, 18.7%

I don't know: 9, 56.2%

I think by chance: 4, 25%

7. Do you believe camaraderie and support from socializing with other patients going through proton therapy is important enough to make it a formal part of the treatment plan?

Number of responses, Percentage of responses

Yes: 11, 68.7%

I am not sure: 5, 31.2%

No: 0, 0%

Specific Comments:

"Some people like me are just loners." "Some people are not comfortable with socializing with others." "Possibly, but spontaneity is better than trying to manage something artificial to the natural camaraderie and support in the dressing room. The dinners appear to fill a void and serve a purpose that may be needed." "I think it is probably more important for those patients receiving treatment who are from out-of-town."

"But a volunteer part of the plan." "But it certainly does help...."

8. Please indicate the importance of each of the following aspects of your treatment by selecting a choice from "Least important" to "Most important."

Least, Somewhat, Important, Most

Your physician: 1 (6%) Least, 1 (6%) Somewhat 5 (31%) Important, 9 (56%)

Interacting with other patients: 0 (0%) Least, 2 (13%) Somewhat, 11 (69%) Important, 3 (19%) Most

Weekly educational seminars: 1 (6%) Least, 4 (25%) Somewhat, 9 (56%) Important, 2 (13%) Most

Getting to know other patients: 0 (0%) Least, 2 (13%) Somewhat, 12 (80%) Important, 1 (7%) Most

Treatment with same patients: 0 (0%) Least, 1 (6%) Somewhat, 12 (75%) Important, 3 (19%) Most

Joke about the treatment: 0 (0%) Least, 3 (19%) Somewhat, 11 (69%) Important, 2 (13%) Most

After hours socializing: 4 (27%) Least, 2 (13%) Somewhat, 8 (53%) Important, 1 (7%) Most

Specific Comments

"I think that for those of us who are from outside of Houston, staying in a strange town, the social aspects of the group are much more important. They fill the need we have as social creatures. Especially for those who have traveled on there own and left friends and family at home." "Travel Distance and Time reduced my participation in the latter activity." "Most Important - Radiation Therapists. These are the people you see five days a week and are performing the "hands on" portion of the treatment. I think it's important one keeps the same group of therapists for the treatment duration." "I lived in the local area, so socializing with other patients on the weekends didn't take on much importance."

9. Please describe your experience in interacting with other patients and indicate if you think it was beneficial (an open ended question).

Specific Comments

"Exhilarating! I met so many different characters." "Just daily camaraderie!" "It was very beneficial." "Enjoyed learning of their interests and about them." "Very important and helpful." "Beneficial not only for me but for the wives." "Similar to the military in similarity of common goals." "Met interesting diverse fun smart positive people." "INTERACTED WITH PATIENTS ONLY AT TREATMENT CENTER." "It was limited but it was good." "Did not anticipate the social aspects. Enjoyed." "Very beneficial for the patient and spouse." "Yes, I do...." "I found interaction very interesting and calming."

10. Do you think treatment centers such as the Proton Therapy Center that provide daily treatment for a protracted period of time should actively facilitate social interaction among its patients?

Number of responses   Percentage of responses
Yes: 12, 75%
Not sure: 3, 18.7%

No: 1, 6.2%
Specific Comments
"I think that this kind of socialization would be good for any medical treatment. The Stigma that people allow themselves to feel can be crushing." "My thoughts are: Don't push it; just let it happen naturally." "Especially if the patients are from out of town."

11. How helpful do you believe the following aspects of treatment would be in terms of improving proton therapy treatment?

Having batches of patients start at the same time and finish at the same time so they could go through as a group. 7% said it would not be helpful, 7% said it may be helpful, 33% were not sure, 40% believed it would be helpful, and 13% believed it would be very helpful.

Keeping the same appointment time to facilitate getting to know the other patients in that time slot: 0% believed it would not help, 19% were not sure, 44% thought it would be helpful, 31% believe it would be very helpful.

Having a staff member to coordinate social events with other patients': 6% said it would not be helpful, 38% said it may be helpful, 38% were not sure, 6% thought it would be very helpful.

Discussing the importance of support from other patients in one of the weekly seminars: 0% said it would not be helpful, 19% said it may be helpful, 6% were not sure, 56% believe it would be very helpful.

Distributing a list of names and phone numbers to all patients and encourage them to contact each other: 0% said it would not be helpful, 6% said it may be helpful, 13% were not sure, 50% said it may be helpful, 31% believe it would be very helpful.

Specific Comments

"Mutual support systems develop naturally; some of us are shy and others are extroverts.... it will work out if one does not organize everything too much. We are still going through an adjustment to the thought of Cancer in the body. We will work through our support without some unknown busy body telling us what to do next. We are grown men."

"I think it would be difficult for groups due to individual desires for different time slots. I needed a time slot that would allow me to go to work; go for a treatment; return to work; and leave for home at a certain time because I van pool. Anyhow, I met some interesting people that I would have never known if they hadn't changed time slots."

Conclusion

The results of this somewhat limited survey clearly indicate the importance patients place on the opportunity to interact and socialize with other patients going through treatment with them. Such social bonding provides health enhancing social support that reduces the fear and anxiety they have associated with their cancer and can help develop a positive and more satisfying attitude among the patients. Treatment centers will be well advised to engage in serious efforts to foster mutual support among their patients. Based on this survey it is likely one of the most important aspects of treatment in terms of overall patient satisfaction. Word of mouth is one of the best ways to market product and services. Treatment centers that facilitate mutual support among its patients will find it has a happy contended group of people spreading the good word about their program.

Recommendations

Proton therapy centers in particular and other health care facilities in general that provide protracted treatment to a large group of patients during the same time frame should seek to facilitate mutual support among their patients by engaging in the following:

1. Schedule to facilitate the development of support

Keep in mind the importance of social support among your patients; it is a key part of the success of your treatment and an even important part of their satisfaction with your facility. Patients should be scheduled in a way that makes it easy for them to get to know each other. This means keeping their appointment time set as opposed to randomly changing it around.

2. Include social functions and special events into the treatment

All of us like going to parties, picnics, and other events with the people we know or are getting to know. Doing this will help your patients to know one another and will foster increased social bonding.

3. Have events where patients and staff can socialize

Forget about the adage "Familiarity breeds contempt" so common in the military. For health care institutions familiarity breeds happiness, satisfaction, and good will, factors that are not only important to your patient's general well being but the bottom line of your facility.

4. Assign responsibility to certain staff for fostering support among the patients

This is not a difficult task nor is it one that will take a great deal of time. All it takes is assigning one employee with overseeing efforts to foster support among your patients.

5. Foster increased communication with your patients

A simple suggestion box does wonders for morale particular when the suggestions from your patients are read and acknowledged.

Appendix C

Where to Receive Proton Therapy

1. Loma Linda University Medical Center
James M Slater Proton Therapy Treatment Center
http://www.protons.com
1+ 800-protons
Loma Linda, CA

2. Francis H Burr Proton Beam Center at Mass. General Hospital
http://www.MassGeneral.org/radiationoncology/BurrProtonCenter.as
px
informationradon@partners.org
617-726-0923, Fax 617-726-6498,Boston , MA

3. Midwest Proton Radiotherapy Institute at Indiana University
http://www.mpri.org866-ITS.MPRI (866-487-6774 Toll free)
812-349-5074 Local
Bloomington, IN

4. Univ. Of Florida Proton Therapy Institute- Shands Medical Center
http://www.FloridaProton.org
877-686-6009, 904-588-1800
Jacksonville, FL

5. M D Anderson Cancer Center-Proton Therapy Center
http://www.mdanderson.org/patient-and-cancer-information/proton-
therapy-center
1+866-632-4PTC, 1+866-632-4782
International patients 713-563-896 1(ask to be transferred to Proton

Therapy info. Line)
Houston, TX

6. Procure Proton Therapy Center- Oklahoma City, OK
http://www.Procure.com/OK
888-847-2640 (US only)
405-773-6767 (International)
Oklahoma City, OK

7. Hampton University Proton Therapy Institute
http://www.Hamptonproton.org
PO Box 6043
Hampton, VA
877-251-6839
info@hamptonproton.org

8. Roberts Proton Therapy Center at University of Pennsylvania
http://www.pennmedicine.org/perelman/proton
800-789-Penn (7366)
Philadelphia, PA

9. CDH Proton Center, A Procure Center
Radiation Oncologist Consultants/Central DuPage Hospital
http://www.procure.com/IL
877-877-5807
Suburban Chicago, IL

10. Rinecker Proton Therapy Center, Munich, Germany
http://mhlclinics.com/rinecker_proton_munich.html
Enquiries: RPTC@mhlhealth.com

11. National Cancer Center/Proton Beam Therapy Center Korea,
Seoul, South Korea
Centers under construction

12. ProCure Proton Therapy Center in partnership with Princeton
Radiation Oncology Group and CentraState Healthcare System,
Somerset, N.J.

13. ProCure Proton Therapy Center in partnership with the Seattle Cancer Care Alliance, Seattle, WA

14. The McLaren Proton Therapy Center, Flint, Michigan
Centers in development

15. Mayo Clinic Proton Beam Therapy Program with locations in Rochester, Minnesota and Phoenix, Arizona

16. The Proton Therapy Center, Knoxville, in partnership with the University of Tennessee Medical Center

17. Proton Institute of New York

Appendix D

Recommended Websites and Books

ProtonBob.com
Protonpals.net
AmercianCancerSocety.com.
NationalCancerInstitute.gov
proton-therapy.org
http://www.hifurx.com (Albert Vorstman, Why should the after effects of some prostate cancer treatments be worse than the disease itself? The Good, The Bad, and The Ugly at, 2011)

Recommended Books on Prostate Cancer

Ralph Blum and Mark Scholz, *Invasion of the Prostate Snatchers*, Other Press: New York, 2011.
Robert J. Marckini, *You Can Beat Prostate Cancer*, 2007 [Paperback]
Fuller Jones, *Prostate Cancer Meets The Proton Beam: A Patient's Experience* [Paperback], 2008.
Karen Demboski and Lois McGuire, *Proton Therapy for Prostate Cancer: More Fun Than We Ever Expected*, Snow In Sarasota Publishing, 2010.
Rick Plummer DMD, *A Prostate Cancer Manifesto: win-win with proton therapy . . . is it right for you*? [Paperback], CreateSpace, 2011.
J. P. Morgan, D.Min., *Faith and Proton Therapy vs. Prostate Cancer* [Paperback], High Pitched Hum Publishing, 2008.
Bradley Hennenfent, *Surviving Prostate Cancer Without Surgery*, Roseville Books, Roseville, IL 2005
Anthony Horan, *The Big Scare: The Business of Prostate Cancer*, SterlingHouse Publisher, Inc., Pittsburg, PA, 2009.
H. Gilbert Welch, Lisa Schwartz, Lisa M. Schwartz, M.D., Steve Woloshin, *Overdiagnosed: Making People Sick in the Pursuit of Health*, Beacon press, Boston. 2011.

Lynn Payer, Disease-Mongers: *How Doctors, Drug Companies, And Insurers Are Making You Feel Sick*, John Wiley, 1992.

Recommended Books on Maintaining Sexual Arousal

Joel Block, Staying Hard: Breakthrough Strategies For Reliable Erections, LuvDoc.com

Rererence Notes

CHAPTER 1

1. Tara Parker-Pope, editor, New York Times Well Blog, On National Public Radio Talk of the Nation, 10-3-11.
2. Albert Vorstman, *Why should the after effects of some prostate cancer treatments be worse than the disease itself?* The Good, The Bad, and The Ugly at http://www.hifurx.com, 2011.
3. Ralph Blum and Mark Scholz, *Invasion Of The Prostate Snatchers: No More Unnecessary Biopsies, Radical Treatment Or Loss Of Sexual Potency,* Other Press: New York, 2011.
4. Anthony Horan, *The Big Scare – The Business of Prostate Cancer,* Sterling House Books, Pittsburg, PA, 2009.

CHAPTER 3

1. Ralph Blum and Mark Scholz, *Invasion Of The Prostate Snatchers: No More Unnecessary Biopsies, Radical Treatment Or Loss Of Sexual Potency,* Other Press: New York, 2011.

CHAPTER 4

1. Ralph Blum and Mark Scholz, *Invasion Of The Prostate Snatchers: No More Unnecessary Biopsies, Radical Treatment Or Loss Of Sexual Potency,* Other Press: New York, 2011.
2. *Minimally Invasive Prostate Cancer Surgery Shows Benefits, Shortcomings,* NCI Cancer Bulletin, vol. 6/no. 20, October 20, 2009
3. Albert Vorstman, *Why should the after effects of some prostate cancer treatments be worse than the disease itself?* The Good, The Bad, and The Ugly at hifurx.com.
4. Bishoff JT, Motley G, Optenberg SA, et al.: *Incidence of fecal and urinary incontinence following radical perineal and retropubic prostatectomy in a national population.* Journal of Urology, 160 (2): 454-8, 1998.
5. Sun M, Lughezzani G, Alasker A, et al.: *Comparative study of inguinal hernia repair after radical prostatectomy, prostate biopsy, transurethral resection of the prostate or pelvic lymph node dissection,* Journal of Urology, 183 (3): 970-5, 2010.

6. Sekita N, Suzuki H, Kamijima S, et al.: *Incidence of inguinal hernia after prostate surgery: open radical retropubic prostatectomy versus open simple prostatectomy versus transurethral resection of the prostate*, International Journal of Urology, 16 (1): 110-3, 2009

7. Savoie M, Kim SS, Soloway MS: *A prospective study measuring penile length in men treated with radical prostatectomy for prostate cancer*, Journal of Urology, 169 (4): 1462-4, 2003.

8. Gontero P, Galzerano M, Bartoletti R, et al.: *New insights into the pathogenesis of penile shortening after radical prostatectomy and the role of postoperative sexual function*, Journal of Urology, 178 (2): 602-7, 2007.

9. McCullough A: *Penile change following radical prostatectomy: size, smooth muscle atrophy, and curve*, Current Urology Reports, 9 (6): 492-9, 2008

10. *Proton Therapy Is Well-Tolerated In Prostate Cancer Patients,* Science Daily, 11-2-09.

11. *Proton therapy may decrease risk for secondary cancers,* reported at the September 2008 50th Annual Meeting American Society for Therapeutic Radiology and Oncology, Posted on HemOncToday.com September 26, 2008.

CHAPTER 5

1. http://health.usnews.com/best-hospitals/rankings/cancer

CHAPTER 7

1. Harold Dawley, *Friendship – How To Make and Keep Friends*, Prentice-Hall: Englewood, New Jersey,1976.

2. Robert Marckini, *You Can Beat Prostate Cancer and You Don't Need Surgery To Do It*, Robert Marckini, 2007 (paperback)

CHAPTER 9

1. Albert Vorstman, *Why should the after effects of some prostate cancer treatments be worse than the disease itself?* The Good, The Bad, and The Ugly at hifurx.com, 2011.

2. Bishoff JT, Motley G, Optenberg SA, et al.: *Incidence of fecal and urinary incontinence following radical perineal and retropubic prostatectomy in a national population,* Journal of Urology, 160 (2): 454-8, 1998)

3. Maeda Y, Høyer M, Lundby L, Norton C., *Faecal incontinence following radiotherapy for prostate cancer: a systematic review.*, Radiotherapy and Oncology, Feb;98(2):145-53, 2011.

4. Feldman HA, Goldstein I , Hatzichristou DG, *Impotence and its medical and psychosocial correlates: Results of the Massachusetts Male Aging Study*, Journal of Urology, 151: 1994; 54-61.

5. Talcott JA, Rossi C, Shipley WU, et al. *Patient-reported long-term outcomes after conventional and high-dose combined proton and photon radiation for early prostate cancer*, Journal of the American Medical Association,303(11):1046-1053, 2010.

6. Hoppe BD, Henderson R, Nichols RC, et al. *Early outcomes following proton therapy for prostate cancer in men 55 years old and younger*, International Journal of Radiation Oncology,Biology, and Physics,78(3):S373-S374, 2010.

7. Robert Marckini, *You Can Beat Prostate Cancer and You Don't Need Surgery To Do It*, Robert Marckini, 2007 (paperback)

8. Victoria Zdrok, Joel Block, Harold. Dawley, *The New Sexually Assertive Woman – A Woman's Guide To Good Sex*, Wellness Institute/Self-Help Books, in press.

9. J. Fontenot. AK Lee, WD Newhauser, *Risk of secondary malignant neoplasms from proton therapy and intensity modulated Xray Therapy for early-stage Prostate cancer*, International Journal of Radiation Oncology, Biology, and Physics, Vol. 74, No. 2, 612-622, 2009.

10. http://www.floridaproton.org/cancer-information/fpt_pr_01262011.html

11. Vargas C, Fryer A, Mahajan C, et al. *Dose-volume comparison of proton therapy and intensity-modulated radiotherapy for prostate cancer*, International Journal of Radiation Oncology,Biology, and Physics, 2, 008;70(3):744-751, 2008.

12. Mendenhall NP, Li Z, Morris CG, et al. *Early GI and GU toxicity in three prospective trials of proton therapy for prostate cancer*, International Journal of Radiation Oncology,Biology, and Physics,75(3):S11-12, 2009.

13. Victoria Zdrok, Joel Block, & Harold Dawley, *The New Sexually Assertive Woman*, Wellness Institute/Self-Help Books, in press.

14. http://www.usatoday.com/news/health/story/health/story/2012-02-01/Study-questions-proton-therapy-for-prostate-cancer/52912536/1

15. http://www.huffingtonpost.com/2012/02/01/proton-therapy-prostate-cancer-side-effects_n_1246873.html

16. http://www.chron.com/news/houston-texas/article/Study-questions-prostate-cancer-therapy-3340528.php

17. David S. Aaronson; Anobel Y. Odisho; Nancy Hills; Rosemary Cress; Peter R. Carroll; R. Adams Dudley; Matthew R. Cooperberg, *Proton Beam Therapy and Treatment for Localized Prostate Cancer: If You Build It, They Will Come,* Arch Intern Med.;172(3):280-283, 2012.

CHAPTER 10
1. Report of the Council on Ethical and Judicial Affairs, Report, American Medical Association, 1-1-08
CHAPTER 11
1. Dana Jennings, *A Rush to the Operating Room That Alters Men's Lives*, The New York Times, 8-30-10.
2. Ralph Blum and Mark Scholz, *Invasion Of The Prostate Snatchers: No More Unnecessary Biopsies, Radical Treatment Or Loss Of Sexual Potency*, Other Press: New York, 2011.
3. Albert Vorstman, *Why should the after effects of some prostate cancer treatments be worse than the disease itself?* The Good, The Bad, and The Ugly at hifurx.com, 2011.
4. Gina Kolata, *Results unproven, robotic surgery wins converts*, The New York Times 2-13-10, http://www.nytimes.com/2010/02/14/health/14robot.html?pagewanted=all
5. Rob Stein , *Doctor-owned centers spark criticism, scrutiny*, The Washington Post, 2-28-11.
6. John Carreyrou and Maurice Tamman, *A Device To Kill Cancer, Lift Revenue*, The Wall Street Journal, 12-7-11.
7. Stephanie Saul, *Profit and Questions on Prostate Cancer Therapy*, New York Times, 2-1-06.
8. Daniel DeNoon,WebMD Poll – How Much Are Doctors Paid, 4-21-11, http://www.webmd.com/healthy-aging/news/20110428/medscape-webmd-poll-how-much-are-doctors-paid
9. Christine Torres, *Robotic surgery extends its reach in health care, hospital marketing*, The Washington Post, 7-16-10.
10. Report of the Council on Ethical and Judicial Affairs, Report, American Medical Association, 1-1-08.
11. 10-7-11 a draft report released by the Health and Human Services Department's Preventive Services Task Force task force, http://www.webmd.com/prostate-cancer/news/20111007/task-force-men-dont-get-psa-test.

12. Gavin Yamey and Michael Wilkes, *Prostate cancer screening – is it worth the pain?* Opinion piece in the 1-18-02 in the Open Forum Section of the San Francisco Chronicle, http://articles.sfgate.com/2002-01-18/opinion/17526729_1_prostate-cancer-screen-healthy-men-prostate-biopsy

13. Gavin Yamey and Michael Wilkes, *The PSA Storm*, BMJ 324 : 431 2-16-02. http://www.bmj.com/content/324/7334/431.full

14. Schröder FH, Hugosson J, Roobol MJ, et al. *Screening and Prostate Cancer Mortality in a Randomized European Study*, New England Journal of Medicine, 2009;360:1320–28. PMID: 19297566

15. Welch HG, Albertsen PC, *Prostate cancer diagnosis and treatment after the introduction of prostate-specific antigen screening: 1986-2005*, Journal of National Cancer Institute 7;101(19):1325-9. Epub 2009 Aug 31.

16. Richard Ablin, Opinion, *The Great Prostate Mistake*, The New York Times, 3-9-10.

17. Otis Brawley, http://www.cnn.com/2011/11/01/opinion/brawley-prostate-cancer-screening/index.html

18. Richard Ablin, *The United States Preventive Task Force Recommendation against Prostate-Specific Antigen Screening – Point*, Cancer Epidemiology, Biomarkers, & Prevention Prev: 21, 3, March 2012.

19. Jeanne Lenzer, Lay campaigners for prostate screening are funded by industry, *British Medical Journal*, 29; 326 (7391): 680., 2003.

20. Ray Moynihan, Iona Heath, and David Henry, *Selling sickness: the pharmaceutical industry and disease mongering*, British Medical Journal, March 29, 2003

CHAPTER 12

1. Richard Ablin, *The Great Prostate Mistake*, The New York Times, 3-9-10.

2. http://news.yahoo.com/u-advisers-no-routine-psa-tests-prostate-cancer-210610161.html

3. Albert Vorstman, Prostate Cancer? Why Radical Surgery/Robotic Prostatectomy Is NOT For You . http://www.urologyweb.com/urology/mens-health/exclusive-medical-reports.html

4. Leonard S Marks and David G Bostwick, Prostate Cancer Specificity of PCA3 Gene Testing: Examples from Clinical Practice, Rev Urol. 2008 Summer; 10(3): 175–181.

5. Phillip Caper, Health *Care Should Be Driven by Mission, Not Money*, <u>CommonDreams.org</u>, December 2, 2009.

www.ingramcontent.com/pod-product-compliance
Lightning Source LLC
Chambersburg PA
CBHW060015210326
41520CB00009B/889